BURN
FAT
FAST

patrick
HOLFORD
& Kate Staples

BURN
FAT
FAST

THE **ALTERNATE-DAY**
LOW-GL DIET PLAN

piatkus

PIATKUS

First published in Great Britain in 2013 by Piatkus
Reprinted 2013

A CIP catalogue record for this book
is available from the British Library.

ISBN 978-0-349-40117-1

Typeset in Minion by M Rules
Printed and bound by CPI Group (UK) Ltd, Croydon, CR0 4YY

Papers used by Piatkus are from well-managed forests
and other responsible sources.

MIX
Paper from
responsible sources
FSC® C104740

Piatkus
An imprint of
Little, Brown Book Group
100 Victoria Embankment
London EC4Y 0DY

An Hachette UK Company
www.hachette.co.uk

www.piatkus.co.uk

Acknowledgements

Sincere thanks to Ann Garry for her help with the recipes, and for tracking volunteers on our Zest4Life programmes to learn what really works. Also, thanks to medical journalist Jerome Burne for his sharp analysis of the current research and helping me unravel 'skinny' genetics; and to my super-efficient manager and assistant Jo Muncaster, for keeping me on target. And a big thanks to my super-enthusiastic and skilful co-author, Kate Staples, for devising the exercise workouts and making sure I do them! Finally, thank you to the team at Little, Brown – Tim Whiting, Jillian Stewart and Jan Cutler, my editors.

About the authors

Patrick Holford BSc, DipION, FBANT, CNHCRP is a leading spokesman on nutrition in the media. He is the author of over 30 books, translated into over 20 languages and selling over a million copies worldwide.

In 1984 he founded the Institute for Optimum Nutrition (ION), an independent educational charity, with his mentor, twice Nobel Prize winner Dr Linus Pauling, as patron. ION has been researching and helping to define what it means to be optimally nourished for the past 25 years and is one of the most respected educational establishments for training nutritional therapists. Patrick was one of the first promoters of the importance of zinc, antioxidants, high-dose vitamin C, essential fats, low-GL diets and B vitamins.

Patrick is Chief Executive Officer of the Food for the Brain Foundation and director of the Brain Bio Centre. He is also an honorary fellow of the British Association of Nutritional Therapy, as well as a registered member of the Complementary and Natural Healthcare Council. See www.patrickholford.com for more information.

Kate Staples has been one of the UK's most prominent names in health, fitness and exercise for more than two decades. As a Great Britain pole vaulter she broke and re-broke a staggering 50 national and Commonwealth records. But it was as Zodiac on the hugely popular UK TV series *Gladiators* that she gained widespread public attention.

Since then Kate has forged an impressive career in a wide variety of health and fitness environments, and holds qualifications in fitness, nutrition and yoga. Her highly successful Adventure Fitness Camps, established with Olympic champion Daley Thompson, operate throughout Britain and overseas. Her aim, through her advice and classes, is to inspire people not only to meet but to exceed their fitness goals. For more information on Kate see www.fitnesscamp.co.uk.

Contents

Introduction – The Three-Day Diet Discovery   xi

1 The History Behind the Alternate-Day Low-GL Diet   1

2 The Low-GL Diet in a Nutshell   22

3 Boosting Your Diet with Exercise   35

4 The Diet and Exercise Workout in Practice   44

5 The Alternate-Day Workout Routines   59

6 The Alternate-Day Low-GL Recipes   77

Recommended Reading   95

Resources   97

Notes   103

Index   106

Introduction – The Three-Day Diet Discovery

Mirror, mirror on the wall, what is the best weight-loss diet of them all? As rates of obesity increase exponentially all over the world, and more and more people struggle to lose weight, the question is what's the easiest, healthiest and most effective way to lose weight and keep it off?

I've been tracking this from the days of low-calorie diets, to the boom of the high-fibre diet in the 1980s, followed by high-protein, low-carb diets in the 1990s, then low-GI (glycemic index) diets based on slow-releasing carbs and, in the last decade, low-GL (glycemic load) diets. Now the latest idea – alternate-day dieting – is rapidly gaining momentum as the fastest and easiest way to burn fat and regain health. The appeal of this kind of dieting is that it involves eating less every other day so that you only have to be on a diet for three days in a week.

To the casual observer all this might look like diet 'fashion', but actually each 'fad' has added something to our understanding of what really makes a difference to weight loss and health.

I am very excited about the discoveries coming from hard

science about alternate-day dieting, because it helps to explain the extraordinary results many people have been achieving with my low-GL diet over the years. Countless people have reported losing a stone (14lb/6.3kg) a month relatively effortlessly and continuously until they have achieved their desired weight by following my tried-and-tested low-GL diet. One man in Ireland lost 7 stone (100lb/44.5kg) in seven months without feeling hungry. Another in the UK lost 9 stone (126lb/57kg) in ten months. These kinds of sustainable results cannot be easily explained just by the simplistic equation of calories in (from food) minus calories out (from exercise).

Something else has to be going on. That 'something' is a total change in your body's metabolism, a kind of biological tune-up, triggered by changes in your genes, which are your body's master control.

We learn in school that you can't change the genes you're born with. This is true, but genes, which are a bit like programs on your computer, can be switched on or off. This is called 'genetic expression', and what's being discovered is that both alternate-day dieting and low-GL diets switch on genes that keep you young, healthy and at the right weight, while switching off genes that trigger ageing and disease. Certain kinds of exercise have the same effect.

I wondered what would happen if I put all three pieces together: eating a low-GL diet but having three moderate fasting days a week and including a compact exercise workout routine.

For those new to my low-GL diet, it stands for 'glycemic load' and is a precise measure of what a food or a meal does to your blood sugar levels. When you follow the diet you consume no more than a certain amount of slow-releasing carbohydrate in a day, measured as GLs. Eating a low-GL diet is the best way to keep your blood sugar level even. If your blood sugar goes too high, the excess is stored as fat, and if it goes too low that's what triggers hunger.

The low-GL diet is based on three rules: (1) eating a little less carbohydrate (and only those that release their sugar slowly); (2) always eating protein with carbs, which further slows down their sugar release; and (3) eating little and often by having three main meals and two snacks daily. Exactly how to do this is explained in Chapter 2.

To create the exercise aspect of my new Alternate-Day Low-GL Diet and Exercise Workout I teamed up with former athlete, celebrity trainer and former Gladiator Kate Staples, whose reputation and results in the world of personal training are second to none.

The latest research has identified how resistance exercise (for building up muscle strength) and interval training triggered the same metabolic and genetic changes that turn you into a fat-burner (more on this in Chapter 3). Kate devised an 8-minute routine to do just this – and this is fully described in Chapter 4 – with online videos so that you can see exactly how to follow it.

Kate's exercise programme doesn't require a huge time input and lots of specialist equipment – quite the opposite, in fact. You really need little more than your body and a few minutes, which can be found by tightening up the order of your day or just setting your alarm clock to go off 15 minutes earlier in the morning.

I then called for volunteers through my weight-loss groups, Zest4Life and my 100% Health Club members to try out the new diet and fitness programme.

Promising results from the start

It's early days with my new diet and fitness approach, but here's some of the feedback we've been receiving from our first wave of Alternate-Day Low-GL Diet and Exercise Workout followers.

'I've been on the plan for almost four weeks and feel fab. I cannot believe how good I feel on the day after the fast day. It's amazing how after the fast days you don't want to binge on processed rubbish – rather you crave the "good" foods!' Kate B.

'I've been doing alternate-fast days with other days of about 55GLs [a higher amount of slow-releasing carbohydrate than you would eat on a regular low-GL diet], sometimes a bit more, based on Patrick's low-GL diet. I've almost abolished my migraine, and I have big improvement in energy levels. Ten days ago I added in resveratrol. I have chronic fatigue syndrome, and although the diet improved things it was very variable on a day-to-day basis. The upshot is a huge improvement in mental energy, and I am now exercising again without major problems, albeit taking it slowly. My joint pain has improved, my skin's improved and I can get out of bed in the morning without it being a major act of willpower. And I've lost 12 pounds [5.4kg] in four weeks, plus 10cm [4in] off my waist. Four weeks ago I would not have believed this was possible.' Dr Eleanor D.

'I'm feeling great on my fasting day! I had a Get Up & Go [shake] breakfast (made with almond milk) and the same for

lunch, and an avocado and tuna salad for dinner. I have to say that I am not nearly as hungry as before and even my daughter has commented that I look good. And I feel very good – very positive with lots of energy! I have also been training, and it has not affected me at all on the fasting day.'
Catherine F.

What I find really encouraging is not just the weight loss but also some almost miraculous health improvements that are being reported. Ellie's story is particularly interesting because she has benefited in a number of ways.

Case study

Ellie, a doctor in Dundee, had tried many diets to lose weight and, more importantly, to combat her chronic fatigue syndrome, migraines, aching joints and, more recently, her menopausal symptoms. Having seen a BBC television programme on alternate-day fasting, and after reading my blog on combining this approach with low-GL eating, she decided to give it a go.

'My main motivation was to regain health. I originally started the low-GL diet while researching and finding out more about the "alternate-day diet" approach. After three days my migraines were hugely better, and although I still have the occasional one, they are far less intense than before. I then decided to do Patrick's ▶

Alternate-Day Diet (which has about 500 calories on alternate days) by having one Get Up & Go shake in the morning and a salad-based meal later in the day, every other day, then following low-GL principles on the days in between.'

Ellie also took the supplements I recommend in Chapter 4.

'On my day off I found I didn't want to eat unhealthy food, so I stuck to about 55–60GLs a day maximum [normally a 'maintenance' level of GLs for people following the regular Holford Low-GL Diet]. Some days I literally found it hard to eat more. Within five days I started to get some real improvements in my energy and arthritic pain but they were a bit variable.'

As the autumn kicked in, Ellie switched to salad and a hot soup and continued to stick to combining protein with carbs at each meal. She has lost almost 2 stone (28lb/12.7kg) so far. She has gained energy and can tolerate exercise again, which used to leave her exhausted and with marked muscle and joint pain, and often fever, in the past.

'I have lost weight before, but hadn't noticed any health benefits for my chronic fatigue syndrome or migraine. One of the joys of this is I have been able, and motivated, to exercise again, even on the fasting days. Exercising on a fasting day doesn't make me feel exhausted. The alternate-day fast also really helps me to understand why I eat. Now I know that in the past I would often eat because I was fatigued. I can now differentiate between eating for physical hunger, whereas before I was eating when I was mentally fatigued.'

I asked her how difficult she found the fasting days.

'The fasting may be challenging for some to start with but it only takes you a couple of days to get into it. Take it a day at a time. When you know you can eat more the next day, it's not so difficult.'

Now, three months on, Ellie's migraines are at their lowest frequency since she was a teenager; her libido has come back; she has much more physical and mental energy and can exercise without feeling exhausted afterwards; she has much less 'need' for sugar or caffeine; her joint pain has completely cleared; the 'awful' cellulite on her arms has completely gone; so too have her menopausal symptoms, with no more hot flushes; and her immune system seems stronger, as she no longer suffers from constant colds and sore throats.

'I have more energy now than I have had in 20 years. Recently, one of my patients said how wonderful it was to see me looking so well. I feel like a new woman. I'd definitely recommend this low-GL diet, alternate-day-fast approach. It's easier than you think and the health benefits for me are certainly worth it.'

If the results above are attractive to you, I recommend you start as soon as possible on my Alternate-Day Low-GL Diet and Exercise Workout. In my experience, it's the fastest way to burn off belly fat and lose weight that is actually practical without requiring an iron will – and it's sustainable. I'll show you how to maintain your rapid weight loss and health improvements once you've achieved your goal.

Before I give you the exact instructions to get you fat-burning, I'd like to give you a bit more background on why this is the way forward and not just some newfangled diet fad.

1

The History Behind the Alternate-Day Low-GL Diet

Before we get into the rules for following my Alternate-Day Low-GL Diet and Exercise Workout, it's worth going back to the beginning to find out about the exciting discoveries that have led me to recommend the combination of alternate-day fasting with a low-GL diet.

Losing weight, and gaining health and energy, is easier to do and more effective when a moderate fast is combined with a low-GL diet than the current alternate-day fasting (ADF) trend of eating a diet that is low in calories (usually about 600 calories – kcal) every other day and eating 'normally' on the other days. I am not convinced that this conventional ADF approach, although effective for some people, is easy enough to follow successfully and sustainably for most people. The only diet that I will support is one that *everyone* can do, in both the short term and the long term, as a way of life, without the pain of hunger or a lack of enjoyment from eating delicious food.

When you understand what's going on inside your cells, I'm sure you'll be convinced – as I am – that my Alternate-Day Low-GL Diet, coupled with specific exercises, represents a major breakthrough in effective weight loss. What's more, as we have seen, the diet also has the additional benefits of helping you to feel great and stay free from disease – adding healthy years to your life. It combines the latest scientifically proven principles for weight loss and health improvement in one simple plan.

Eat less, live longer

Back in the 1980s, when I founded the Institute for Optimum Nutrition, I was intrigued by the research of a charismatic, if somewhat eccentric, professor of gerontology (the study of ageing), Roy Walford. He was the first person to show that you could extend the lifespan of animals by up to 50 per cent by feeding them a very low-calorie diet. It also worked in primates, so he had every reason to believe it would work in humans too. He then became the first human guinea pig. Later, he enrolled others to follow his daily calorie-restriction, or CR, regime (they would later become known as 'CRonies'), eating usually between 1,200 and 1,500 calories a day. He, and later researchers, were able to show a number of changes in the body. The mitochondria, which are the energy factories in cells, started to work better, protein production improved and various markers for health, such as blood pressure, blood sugar balance and weight, all improved with CR.

A more recent example of the benefits of CR was a study where 11 people with diabetes were put on a 600-calorie diet for eight weeks. One thing to note is that if you are diabetic your pancreas stops working properly and no longer produces insulin. Seven out of the 11 people were no longer diabetic at the end of the study and there was evidence that their pancreatic cells had returned to life and were producing insulin again.[1]

The only drawback to this magical transformation is that it's almost impossible for us humans to follow such a low-calorie diet. You have to be a fanatic, ready to put up with feeling cold because you are not taking in many calories and prepared for living on the edge of hunger for most of the time. Even then, it's not absolutely certain that you will actually live any longer, because we don't have a group of people who have been doing this for long enough to find out; however, a long-running study found that primates benefited substantially from the diet, making it even more likely that humans would too.

Exactly why CR works wasn't known at the time that Walford was first studying the very low-calorie diet and lifespan, but the prevalent theory was that if you 'burn' less food you make fewer oxidants, which are the body's equivalent of exhaust fumes, and which produce an ageing effect. By taking in all the necessary nutrients, vitamins, minerals, antioxidants and so on, with fewer calories, the body could be super-efficient – in other words, a lean, mean fighting machine. Walford also found that his CR mice were more physically active, and so he advocated daily exercise plus low calories as the way to proceed if you wanted to live longer and be healthier.

Switching on the 'skinny' genes

Sadly, Dr Roy Walford died young in 2004 from respiratory failure as a complication of amyotrophic lateral sclerosis, a disease that he had been fighting for years, so he was not able to discover the next quantum leap in the understanding of the effect of CR on the body or, more precisely, on the genes.

Back in 2007, geneticist Professor Cynthia Kenyon, of the University of California, considered what effect CR was having on gene activity. To test this she used the genetic researcher's 'lab rat' – tiny roundworms known as *Caenorhabditis elegans*, which are just a millimetre long – and put them on low-calorie diets.

She found that one gene in particular was switched off by the CR diet. To her big surprise, it was one that normally made more insulin available. Even more of a surprise was the finding that switching the insulin gene off switched on another gene that controlled a cascade of extensive cell-repair processes. By tinkering with these genes she was able to breed some worms that lived for twice their normal 20-day lifespan. Recently, using more sophisticated techniques, Kenyon has been able to genetically engineer a strain of *C. elegans* that lives healthily and actively for an astonishing 144 days. That's the human equivalent of 450 years!

Discovering this genetic mechanism had opened the way to

looking at healthy lifestyle changes in a much more focused way. It has also revolutionised ageing research, according to Jeff Holly, Professor of Clinical Sciences at Bristol University. 'Ten years ago we thought ageing was probably the result of a slow decay, a sort of rusting [oxidation],' he says, 'but Cynthia [Kenyon] has shown that it's not about wear and tear but instead it is controlled by genes. That opens the possibility of slowing it down.' The connection to such research and my low-GL diet is that my diet also avoids sharp increases in insulin, so it is achieving a similar result to the very low-calorie diets used by Kenyon and Walford.

Insulin is the ageing hormone

The key to both slowing ageing and burning fat is keeping the amount of insulin in your bloodstream down. (Insulin is released into the bloodstream whenever your blood sugar level goes up.) Dr Kenyon's discoveries about what the genes in her long-lived worms were doing showed that too much insulin was switching 'bad' genes on and 'good' genes off. 'We jokingly called the first gene the Grim Reaper,' she said, 'because when it's on, which is the normal state of affairs, [the worms'] lifespan is fairly short.'

The second gene had such a remarkable effect on the worms' health that it was quickly nicknamed 'Sweet Sixteen', because it reduced the worms' 'age', turning them into the equivalent of svelte teenagers. Kenyon had stumbled on a genetic Shangri-La – the fictional valley where people barely aged, and stayed slim and healthy.

Fortunately, humans have an equivalent gene to Sweet

Sixteen, called Foxo. Switching that gene on has a number of remarkable effects. 'Your supply of natural antioxidants goes up, damping down damaging oxidants,' says Kenyon. 'There's a boost to compounds that make sure the skin and muscle-building proteins are working properly, the immune system becomes more active in fighting infection and genes that are active in cancer get turned off.'

What surprised many is that the research clearly implicated high insulin as being a key player in ageing and weight control, and very possibly in diabetes, heart disease and cancer. One clear message was that keeping your insulin levels to a minimum, which is exactly what a low-GL diet achieves, could be a recipe for staying slim, young and healthy. It's what I've been recommending for years. It's also what Kenyon herself is now doing since she found that after giving her super-centenarian worms just one drop of glucose they rapidly became wrinkly and then died young. She now keeps her carbohydrate intake low and eats lots of vegetables.

High blood sugar, which triggers insulin in the body, means that the Grim Reaper gene stays on, so the Foxo gene is never activated. So to ensure that Foxo is activated in our body we need to retain an even blood sugar level – and that is the aim of the low-GL diet.

The IGF factor, cancer and Ecuadorian dwarves

Although meat, and especially dairy products, don't have a high GL, in other words they don't raise your blood sugar much, they do tell the body to release an insulin-like growth hormone called IGF-1. This hormone makes baby cells grow fast, so it's perfect when you're a newborn infant. But IGF-1 also switches on the Grim Reaper genes that age you and stop you burning fat. Whereas an Atkins-type high-meat/milk-protein diet may work for short-term weight loss, I don't advocate them for those wanting to achieve optimal health. In fact, meat and milk consumption is strongly linked to an increased risk of many diseases, especially cancer. A review of 23 studies carried out by the National Cancer Institute reported that 19 of them show a positive association between dairy intake and prostate cancer. The same is true for breast cancer and also colorectal cancer, which is also strongly linked to meat consumption, especially red and processed meat.

This association is made even more real by a rather unusual community of dwarves living in Ecuador, who are cancer-free. They are missing the part of the Grim Reaper gene that controls IGF-1, of which they are, in effect, deficient. This has an upside, in that they remain cancer-free. The downside is that they grow to only 4 feet (1.2m) tall, because IGF-1 is needed for growth, but they are also less likely to suffer from heart disease or obesity.[2] The more dairy products you eat, the more IGF-1 you produce.

Insulin and its connection to ill health

It looks plausible that the largest of our chronic killers and the epidemic of obesity might have a common origin, linked by an excess of insulin. As well as controlling blood sugar, raised insulin triggers an increase in cholesterol production in the liver. It also makes the walls of blood vessels contract so that blood pressure goes up. This action stimulates the release of fats called triglycerides, which are linked to a raised risk of heart disease and diabetes.

Contrary to popular opinion, eggs, although high in cholesterol, do not raise blood cholesterol. Sugar and refined carbohydrates, on the other hand, raise insulin levels and cause increases in cholesterol, blood pressure, blood sugar and blood fats. It's the toast that goes with the eggs, and not the eggs themselves, that is the problem. Our modern-day, high-carb diet is a recipe for disaster.

In 2010, Harvard geneticist Dr Kevin Struhl made a surprising discovery when he found that 300 genes linked with tumour growth were also connected with obesity, heart disease and diabetes. Some of those genes affect insulin.[3] 'I was shocked when we found this,' he says. 'People had suspected there might be an underlying link between all these diseases but this puts it on molecular footing.' Current research suggests that it is insulin that drives obesity, not the other way around.

The great news for you is that the diet I recommend for rapidly burning off unwanted fat is exactly the diet that can halve your risk of today's chronic killer diseases. And that's one of the main reasons this diet is alternate-day *and* low-GL.

Chromium and cinnamon lower insulin

Although it appears that the holy grail of health is to lower insulin levels – the cornerstone of a low-GL diet – another way is to improve your *sensitivity* to insulin. The docking port for insulin, the insulin receptor, is dependent on the mineral chromium, but this is often deficient in today's diet of refined food. The process of refining sugar, for example, removes 98 per cent of the chromium contained in the raw sugar. Also, the more sugar and carbs you eat the more chromium you need. Without sufficient chromium for the insulin receptor to work efficiently, you become increasingly insensitive to insulin, known as 'insulin resistance'.

Supplementing extra chromium, especially for those with insulin resistance or diabetes, has remarkable effects, as the following study illustrates. Diabetic patients were given 500mcg of chromium per day for eight months. There was a major improvement in both fasting blood sugar levels and blood sugar levels after meals, as a consequence of improved insulin sensitivity.[4]

A systematic review in the top diabetes journal, *Diabetes Care*, concludes that 'chromium supplementation improved glycosylated haemoglobin (HbA1c) levels and fasting glucose.'[5] When your blood sugar goes too high, which triggers insulin release, red blood cells (haemoglobin) become sugar-damaged (glycosylated), so having a low level of what's called HbA1c is very good news.

In a more recent study, healthy, overweight women were given chromium or a placebo for eight weeks. Those on the chromium ate less, felt less hungry, craved fat less and also lost more weight than those taking the placebos.[6] Of course, this makes eating a low-GL or low-calorie diet easier.

So too does eating, or supplementing, the spice cinnamon, as seen in the studies below:

- People with pre-diabetes who were given a cinnamon extract (cinnulin) for 12 weeks had reduced blood sugar levels, blood pressure, body-fat percentage and oxidation.[7]

- Thirty-nine diabetic patients were given cinnamon extract for four months. It was found that there was a substantial reduction in their post-meal blood sugar levels and a 10 per cent reduction in fasting blood sugar levels.

- Volunteers who were given rice pudding, with or without cinnamon, found that those given 3g cinnamon produced less insulin after the meal. That's about ½ teaspoon a day, equivalent in power to 150mg of the cinnamon extract, cinnulin. (Cinnulin is 20 times more potent, mg per mg, than the spice cinnamon, because it concentrates the active ingredient, called MCHP.)

In my experience, the combination of chromium (400mcg) and cinnulin (150mg) is a winning formula.

So far we have learnt that cutting calories, eating a low-GL diet and supplementing cinnamon and chromium can all help you to lose weight, prevent and reverse disease and switch on anti-ageing genes. Now let's look at how limiting calories can work in practice so that it is possible to reduce your calorie intake without feeling discomfort and constant hunger.

The alternate-day discovery

A low-GL diet looks like a powerful way to keep insulin at a healthy level, but if we also want to restrict calories, there is another way to get the benefits without being condemned to a permanent state of semi-starvation. The principle is ridiculously simple: fast every other day. That's it. You eat less for one day and eat as much as you like the next. Fast for another day, then eat normally, and so on.

Of course, there are variations and guidelines depending on the fasting diet you follow. Most people eat something on the 'down' day, as it is called: usually up to 50 per cent of the calories you'd normally have, depending on how much or how quickly you want to lose weight. In animal studies it seems you need at least 20 per cent fewer calories than your basic metabolic needs to trigger a positive change in metabolism and genetic expression.

In 2003 Dr Mark Mattson, a neuroscientist at the National Institute on Aging, discovered that rats put on the every-other-day schedule did just as well as their relatives on the gruelling CR diet first proposed by Dr Walford back in the 1980s.[8]

This alternate-day approach has much wider potential health benefits too. A number of researchers have discovered that its effect on genes can also help with various health problems:

- In one small study, asthma patients lost 8 per cent of their bodyweight, and with it they saw a dramatic drop in levels of inflammation and damaging oxidants; symptoms of wheezing and shortness of breath both greatly improved.[9]

- In another study, overweight patients lost weight more easily than usual and produced greater amounts of a protein called adiponectin, which reduces insulin resistance and damps down inflammation.[10]

- In an animal study, alternate-day dieting reduced inflammation and also increased the level of sirtuin, nicknamed the 'skinny gene', because it initiates metabolic changes that assist weight control.[11]

The correct strategy

There is still a lot of research going on – and needed – to find the winning formula. Some researchers are testing severe calorie restriction one day a week, whereas others are studying alternate-day modified fasting. The best results so far appear to be achieved fasting three days a week.

My Alternate-Day Low-GL Diet is made up of three days of modified fasting, which means that on three days each week you will eat fewer calories, around 800, of low-GL foods. These fast days are followed by feast days, where you continue to eat low-GL foods but you will be allowed a higher quantity than you would if you were following my standard Low-GL diet.

What about the role of fats?

You may be wondering whether eating foods that are higher in fats on your non-fasting day will make a difference to whether you lose weight or not. A study by Monica Klempel at the University of Illinois examined the difference between eating a low-fat diet on one day and eating a high-fat diet the next day. Both groups lost significant amounts of weight (a 4.8 per cent reduction), 11lb (5kg) of body fat and 2¾in (7cm) off their waist in the two weeks of the study. They also had a significant decrease in cholesterol and triglycerides. But there was little difference between those dieters who ate low-fat foods and those who ate high-fat foods the day after.[12]

This is not so surprising, because the key factor that switches on the 'skinny' genes is the release of insulin, which is achieved with low-GL eating, *not* low fat. The research that needs to be done next is examining the difference between a low-GL diet and a high-GL diet on the non-fasting days.

A further study was made by the same team. This time they used a liquid low-calorie diet of about 1,000 calories taken as a shake with one day of fasting a week. They reported an approximate 8lb (about 4kg) weight loss and 6lb (2.8kg) fat loss over eight weeks. Cholesterol levels in the subjects dropped by 8 per cent, and so did heart rate, glucose, insulin and homocysteine – all good signs of significant health improvement.[13]

My simple and straightforward three-day-a-week diet is based on all the ground-breaking research above, but because it is based on GLs rather than simply calories – although I do restrict them on the fast days – you have all the benefits with none of the downsides. For three days a week you eat less, but because you will be following my low-GL diet principles you won't have to go hungry. On the other days you follow my GL principles but you have more leeway. So you don't have to be a saint every day. My low-GL diet is based on proper meals with real food, giving you food that you will find satisfying and enjoyable to eat, not restricting you to foods that leave you feeling hungry and wanting to snack unhealthily throughout the day. All the guidelines, including what to eat on your fasting days and the days in between, are provided in the following chapters.

Are there any downsides?

At this point you might be wondering if this way of eating might make you feel mentally or physically tired. This was tested in an animal study and no evidence was found of a lack of mental energy. The alternate-day fasting did, however, improve insulin sensitivity, which, apart from being good for health, may also be the reason why the animals had no decline in mental energy. This is because improved insulin sensitivity means a better ability to turn blood sugar into energy.[14] Most people report having more, not less, mental and physical energy.

Furthermore, as we have seen, animal studies consistently show a slowing down of the ageing process and with it a reduction in the risk of the chronic diseases of ageing, including heart disease.[15]

Not all the news is good, however. Chronic alternate-day dieting in animals (which is not what my diet recommends), although prompting weight loss, prolonging life, reducing metabolic risk factors for diabetes and cardiovascular diseases, and reducing the prevalence of age-related diseases, has also shown some potential harm for heart-muscle function in rats in the long-term, according to Mattson's team at the National Institute on Ageing, in Baltimore, Maryland.[16] So, just how long you should be on this kind of regimen is yet to be clarified.

Among CRonies (you may remember that these are people following low-calorie diets over several years) there is evidence of reduced bone mass, reduced fertility and menstrual abnormalities, as well as feeling cold, and having a lack of body fat.

There is also the risk of becoming obsessed with what you eat and encouraging an eating disorder to develop. You are unlikely to encounter these kinds of problems with short-term low-calorie diets but, conversely, short-term restriction is hardly likely to lengthen your lifespan. That's why it is more important to find a long-term solution that you can stick to that controls your weight, keeps you healthy and lengthens your life, and this is what my Alternate-Day Low-GL Diet achieves.

Another concern about low-calorie diets is that the body 'fights back' by slowing down metabolism to conserve body weight: you think you're dieting; your body thinks you're starving. I know of no evidence that this happens with my Alternate-Day Low-GL Diet, and Kate Staples has included a cardio workout on the fast day, which speeds up your metabolic rate in any case. The combination of a low-GL diet – which has been shown not to cause the same rebound drop in metabolism found with low-calorie diets – and aerobic exercise should certainly prevent any rebound drop in metabolism.

My advice is to use this Alternate-Day Diet to bring your weight down and restore health, then to follow a basic low-GL diet with one fasting day a week if necessary. Most people find this way of eating becomes their way of life. Jennifer, for example, lost nearly 5 stone (70lb/31.7kg).

'It's changed my life. I no longer crave sweet foods. The recipes give me constant energy. I will never go back to eating any other way.'

I hear this feedback from low-GL dieters again and again.

It's easier than you think

At first sight all this might sound quite hard to do, but in reality it's much easier than you think, as many people have told me. One volunteer, a doctor from Scotland, said, 'Take it a day at a time. If you know you can eat more the next day it's not so difficult.'

This is borne out by the research. In a study of 16 obese people, participants quickly adapted to the alternate-day fasting regime and, by the second week of an eight-week diet, they were not feeling significantly hungry on the fasting days. They lost close to 6kg (13lb) and 1½in (4cm) from the waist eating about 500 calories on the fasting days.[17] Their LDL cholesterol also dropped by 25 per cent.

Many of our volunteers report that on the feast days they just didn't feel particularly hungry.

Case study

Wendy, who lost 6 stone (84lb/38kg) and reversed her diabetes, says:

'My "down" days were very easy to do and I always felt very well at the end of them. I quickly noticed that hunger comes in waves, and if I can ride each wave then I come out the other side OK. By 5.00pm I had no hunger at all for the rest of the evening. On my "up" days I had no desire to eat any extra.'

This is, of course, an added benefit for this approach, because you naturally won't compensate as much as you'd think on the non-fasting days. Overall, then, your calorie intake goes down.

Exercise plus alternate-day low-GL eating: the winning formula

The secret is to combine low-GL principles with alternate-day eating and the right kind of exercise. As we have seen, exercise has been shown to trigger gene 'switching' similar to calorie restriction. In animals, exercise promotes the sirtuin genes associated with upgrading the energy-producing capacity of cells, which means more fat-burning capacity.[18] But it's not just animals who benefit. In a 12-week study, obese people were put on either an alternate-day fast, or on an exercise regime, or both. Those combining alternate-day fasting with exercise lost twice as much weight (6kg/13lb) as those just doing alternate-day fasting (3kg/6.6lb). Those just doing the exercise lost very little (1kg/2.2lb).[19]

Will you feel like exercising on the fasting days? In the study mentioned above the volunteers continued exercising (6,500 steps a day) on the fasting days without any problem. I often hear from people who say their energy levels are much higher and that they enjoy exercising on the fast days.

FAQs about my Alternate-Day Low-GL approach

Q What are the advantages of the alternate-day approach compared with the more commonly used two days fasting per week?

A Most of the alternate-day research showing benefits in health and weight loss were on alternate-day low-calorie diets, *not* just fasting for two days a week. I am not convinced that two fast days alone can really achieve what we are achieving with three fast days, and most people find these extremely doable.

Q Why are the fast days recommended in this book 800 calories whereas other approaches are 500 or 600 calories?

A Although some studies that focus only on calories, and that use fewer calories than my diet, have shown substantial benefits, this kind of regime is hard to follow and to sustain. Other studies show that either halving calorie intake (a moderately active woman's calorie needs are about 2,000 calories, for example) or having 20 per cent fewer calories overall, which is what my diet achieves averaged over the week, switches genes and metabolism to fat-burning.

Q If the diet is based on GLs, why are you counting fast-day calories instead of just GLs?

A Although switching on skinny genes seems to be based on insulin levels, which would favour just continuing GLs, quite a lot of the research to date has been based on calories, so the Alternate-Day Low-GL Diet makes sure you achieve both criteria on the fast days.

Q What are the benefits of 'controlling' food on feast days?
A Stabilising your blood sugar, and reversing insulin resistance, takes time and leads to fewer food and sugar cravings, and more ability to burn fat. Rather than taking two steps forward on the fast days, followed by two steps back by eating anything on the feast days, following low-GL principles on the feast days keeps you making good progress towards health, weight loss and blood sugar control.

Q Why are three meals and one snack included, whereas other approaches advocate a maximum of two meals with larger gaps?
A By eating little and more often you reduce the amount of insulin your body has to produce – and it's insulin, or lack of it, that switches on the skinny genes.

Q Will I feel hungry on fast days?
A Most people report very little hunger. You may have some hungry phases in the first couple of days. If you resist, you may find they go away. You'll start to learn the difference between real hunger and craving carbohydrates because your blood sugar level is low.

Q I am new to low-GL, can I start immediately with the Alternate-Day Low-GL Diet?
A Yes, you can. The most important thing to start with is getting used to eating low-GL foods. You may want to take

▶

a week to familiarise yourself with eating in this way, then start the fast days in your second week.

Q How long can I stay on the Alternate-Day Diet?
A As long as you need to. Once you achieve your desired weight and health you can continue to have one fast day a week, the remainder being low-GL at your best 'maintenance' level, see page 55.

Q Is it suitable for everyone?
A Almost, but if you have diabetes, although this way of eating is very good, you need to be careful not to leave too long between meals. Tread carefully, ideally with the guidance and support of a healthcare practitioner. You may find your need for medication changes, so it's good to inform your doctor that you are trying a low-GL diet. (My book *Say No to Diabetes* has a precise programme for both people with type-1 and type-2 diabetes. This is a more appropriate way to apply low-GL diet principles if you are diabetic.)

In Chapter 2 I'm going to explain the principles of low-GL eating in a nutshell so that you know how to keep your blood sugar even. With even blood sugar there will be no energy dips, sugar cravings or irresistible hunger pangs. If you are new to low-GL, this is a great place to start. I recommend familiarising yourself with the principles of how to keep your blood sugar stable. In fact, many people have found that adopting low-GL first, for at least 3–4 weeks, is a great introduction to the Alternate-Day Diet.

In Chapter 3, former Gladiator Kate Staples will explain the principles behind her alternate-day fat-burning exercise routine. Kate has devised an 8-minute strength-training routine that builds lean muscle, keeping you both trim and fit, which you do on alternate days.

We will then get down to the exact instructions, with eating plans, recipes and exercises to turn you into an overnight fat-burner!

2

The Low-GL Diet
in a Nutshell

For those new to low-GL, it stands for low glycemic load and is a way to keep your blood sugar level even. When your blood sugar level goes high, insulin is released into the blood to take the glucose (sugar) out. Some of it goes to the brain and the muscles, but if you've eaten more than you need, the remainder goes to the liver, which turns it into fat and stores it in the nearest place possible, starting with your waist. Insulin is, therefore, the fat-storing hormone. Once insulin kicks in, blood glucose levels drop and this triggers hunger and the release of stress hormones to get you ready to go hunting for more food. Your appetite, sugar and carb cravings kick in as a result.

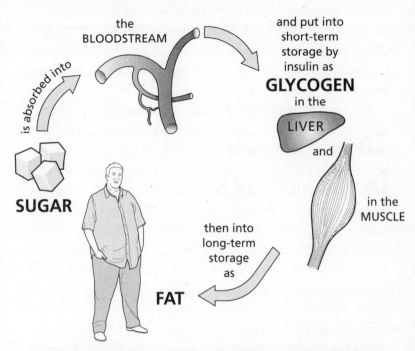

How the body stores energy as fat The body runs on sugar (glucose) and insulin converts any extra into glycogen, which is stored in the mucles and the liver. If glycogen stores are full the body converts glucose into fat, our long-term energy storage.

The importance of sensitivity to insulin

The more blood sugar highs (followed by lows) you have, the more blunted or 'deaf' the receptor sites become for recognising insulin inside the arteries and cells. In time you become what is known as insulin-resistant, because you have increasingly less sensitivity to insulin. Your body then has to produce even more insulin to achieve the desired effect of lowering blood glucose. This is bad news, because it switches off the anti-ageing genes and switches on the Grim Reaper genes. You also start getting 'rebound' blood sugar lows when the insulin finally kicks in.

The symptoms of low blood sugar include poor concentration, irritability, nervousness, depression, sweating, headaches and digestive problems. But most of all you feel tired and hungry. If you refuel with fast-energy-releasing high-GL carbohydrates such as sugary snacks or bread-based foods, you then cause your blood sugar to rise rapidly. Your body doesn't need that much sugar, so it dumps the excess into storage as fat. Your blood sugar level then dips down to low again. This is how you enter the vicious cycle of yo-yoing blood sugar that leads to tiredness, weight gain and carbohydrate cravings.

An estimated three in every ten people have impaired ability to keep their blood sugar level stable. If this is you, the result, over the years, is that you are likely to become increasingly fatter and more lethargic. If you can control your blood sugar levels, the result is stable weight and constant energy.

I have been advocating a low-GL diet for over a decade and have had people reporting to me that they have lost 15 pounds (7kg) in a month without going hungry. Thousands of people have benefited from following my low-GL principles, reversing diabetes and heart disease, regaining health and losing weight. By adding the 'alternate day' principles you can achieve an even better, and faster, weight loss.

High-fat, high-protein diets are not healthy

There are two extremes for achieving a low-GL meal. One, first advocated by the late Dr Robert Atkins, is to avoid carbohydrates, eating high protein and fat instead. This kind of diet is very high in meat and dairy products. The other, which is preferable for reasons I will explain, is to have some carbohydrates, but only those that release their sugar content slowly, and to always eat them with protein; for example, the main sugar in berries is xylose, which has a very low GL, and, if you eat them with seeds high in protein, such as pumpkin or chia seeds, the net effect is very low GL.

One reason I prefer this approach is that meat, and especially dairy products, actually raise a type of insulin called insulin-like growth factor, or IGF-1. As I explained in Chapter 1, this, like too much insulin, is bad news.

The three golden GL rules

The best way to achieve stable blood sugar balance is to control the glycemic load – or GL – of your diet. The reason I focus on the carbohydrate content of foods is that the other two main food types – fat and protein – don't have any appreciable effect on blood sugar. In fact, I recommend you eat some fat and protein with your carbohydrate, because this will further lessen the effect the carbohydrate has on your blood sugar, thereby lowering the GL of the meal. You'll find my menus are balanced to give a protein food, such as fish, with a carbohydrate-rich food, such as rice.

For balancing your blood sugar, there are only three rules:

Rule 1 Eat 40GLs a day to lose weight, 60GLs to maintain it

Rule 2 Eat carbohydrate with protein

Rule 3 Graze, don't gorge

The third rule means eating little and often. So always eat breakfast, lunch and supper – and introduce a snack midmorning and midafternoon. This way you'll provide your body with a constant and even supply of fuel, which means you'll experience fewer food cravings.

Understanding the glycemic load

The glycemic load is a measurement that tells you to what degree the carbohydrate content of a given food will raise blood sugar levels. Raised blood sugar levels, as we have seen, lead to weight gain. If it is a low-GL food, it will not affect weight gain; a high-GL food, on the other hand, will cause you to put on weight. The glycemic load (GL) is based the glycemic index (GI). Put simply, the glycemic index of a food tells you whether the carbohydrate in the food is fast- or slow-releasing. It's a 'quality' measure. It doesn't tell you, however, how much of the food is carbohydrate.

Carbohydrate points, or grams of carbohydrate, tell you how much of the food is carbohydrate, but they don't tell you what the particular carbohydrate does to your blood sugar. It's a 'quantity' measure. The glycemic load of a food is the quantity times the quality. It's the best way of telling you whether you'll gain weight if you choose a particular food.

Here are some examples of high- and low-GL carbohydrates to give you an idea of which kinds of foods to choose, and why the carbohydrate foods in the recipes in this book have been chosen. Ideally, you want to eat 5GLs for a snack and 7–10GLs for the carbohydrate portion of a main meal. The low-GL foods are shown in bold, the moderate-GL in ordinary text, and the high-GL in italics.

Food	Serving looks like	GL
FRUIT		
Blueberries	**1 large punnet (600g)**	**5**
Apple	**1 small (100g)**	**5**
Grapefruit	**1 small**	**5**
Apricot	**4 apricots**	**5**
Pear	**1 pear**	**5**
Plum	**4 plums**	**5**
Banana	1 small banana	10
Raisins	*20 raisins*	*10*
Dates	*2 dates*	*10*
STARCHY VEGETABLES		
Pumpkin/squash	**1 large serving (185g)**	**7**
Carrot	**1 large (158g)**	**7**
Beetroot	**2 small**	**5**
Boiled potato	3 small potatoes (60g)	5
Sweet potato	1 sweet potato (120g)	10
Baked potato	1 baked potato (120g)	10
French fries	*10 fries*	*10*

▶

Food	Serving looks like	GL
GRAINS, BREADS, CEREALS		
Quinoa (cooked)	**65g (⅔ cup)**	**5**
Pearl barley (cooked)	**75g**	**5**
Brown basmati rice (cooked)	1 small serving (70g)	5
White rice (cooked)	*½ serving (66g)*	*10*
Couscous (soaked)	*½ serving (66g)*	*10*
Rough oatcakes	**2–3 oatcakes**	**5**
Pumpernickel-style rye bread	**1 thin slice**	**5**
Wholemeal bread	1 thin slice	5
Bagel	*¼ bagel*	*5*
Puffed rice cakes	*1 rice cake*	*5*
White pasta (cooked)	1 small serving (78g)	10
BEANS AND LENTILS		
Soya beans	**3½ cans**	**5**
Pinto beans	**1 can**	**5**
Lentils	**1 large serving (200g, cooked)**	**7**
Kidney beans	**1 large serving (150g, cooked)**	**7**
Chickpeas	**1 large serving (150g, cooked)**	**7**
Baked beans	1 large serving (150g)	7

For a complete list of foods and their GL score, check out my free GL counter at www.holforddiet.com.

Breaking the sugar habit

The taste for concentrated sweetness is often acquired in childhood. If sweet things are used as a reward or to cheer someone up, they become emotional comforters. The best way to break the habit is to avoid concentrated sweetness in the form of sugar, sweets, sweet desserts, dried fruit and neat fruit juice. Dilute fruit juice with water and get used to eating fruit instead of having a dessert. Sweeten breakfast cereals with fruit, and have fruit instead of sweet snacks. If you gradually reduce the sweetness in your food, you will get used to the taste.

Sugar alternatives

Beware of switching to natural sugars such as honey or maple syrup, as these still cause a rapid increase in blood sugar. Artificial sweeteners are not so great either. Some have been shown to have harmful effects on health, and all perpetuate a sweet tooth. One of the best sugar alternatives is xylitol, a vegetable sugar that has a very low GL. It tastes much the same as regular sugar but has little effect on blood sugar. Nine teaspoons of xylitol, for example, have the equivalent effect of just one teaspoon of regular sugar or honey. Another low-GL sweetener is agave syrup. You will find these two sweeteners used in some recipes. Both should be used sparingly, however, so that your taste buds can get used to less sweet foods.

A model low-GL meal

Here's a simple way to apply my low-GL principles to give you healthy, well-balanced and satisfying lunches and dinners. Protein should make up one-quarter of your meal. Protein foods include: fish, meat, eggs or tofu, or a serving of beans or lentils (soya, pinto, borlotti and lentils have the most protein). Another quarter of your plate should have starchy carbohydrates, such as brown rice, potatoes, wholegrain pasta, wholemeal bread, quinoa and couscous. You can also include pulses such as kidney beans, butter beans or chickpeas, split peas or lentils as your carb portion, because they contain carbs and protein, so this further lowers the GL of your meal. Half your plate should be fresh low-carbohydrate vegetables or salad. Here's what it looks like on your plate.

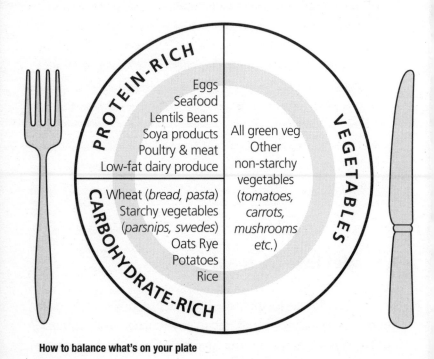

How to balance what's on your plate

Protein options

For optimal health, the message is to eat more vegetable protein and fish, and less red meat and dairy. Experiment with foods such as tofu – which you can buy marinated and ready to toss into stir-fries or salads. The protein-rich grain quinoa is easy to cook – just add double the quantity of water or vegetable stock and gently simmer for 15 minutes. Lentils, chickpeas and beans can be enjoyed in pâtés or dips (such as hummus) and can also be added to stews and pasta sauces for some high-fibre protein (buy ready-to-eat beans in tins, or soak and cook your own dried beans).

Fish is easy to cook: steam, grill or bake with lemon and herbs. Tinned fish is also a cheap and easy way to add lean protein to a meal. Add some anchovies to a pasta sauce, for example, or mix wild salmon with cooked potatoes and onions to make a tasty fishcake (bind with an egg, add some seasoning and dust with flour or cornmeal before grilling).

Balancing carbohydrates

As you are probably beginning to realise by now, not all carbs are created equal. For optimal health, eat slow-releasing carbohydrates – that is, those with the lowest GL score. Here are some examples of starchy carbohydrates (in other words, those that contain more sugar) with a glycemic load of 7 (7GLs). The reason I give a total of 7GLs is that half a plate of vegetables or salad averages 3 GLs. So 7 + 3 = 10GLs, which is the maximum you should eat in a meal on your fast days. On your feast days you can increase the starchy carb portion to a maximum of 10GLs, as shown below, although many people find a 7GL portion suffices.

Starchy carb	7GLs looks like	10GLs looks like
Pumpkin/squash	1 large serving (186g)	Double a regular serving (266g)
Carrot	1 large (158g)	2 regular (266g)
Swede	1 regular serving (150g)	1 large serving (214g)
Quinoa	1 regular serving (120g)	1 large serving (188g)
Baked beans	1 large serving (150g)	Double a regular serving (214g)
Lentils	1 large serving (175g)	Double a regular serving (300g)
Kidney beans	1 large serving (150g)	Double a regular serving (214g)
Pearl barley	1 small serving (95g)	1 regular serving (136g)
Wholemeal pasta	½ serving (85g)	1 large serving (112g)
White pasta	⅓ serving (66g)	1 small serving (78g)
Brown rice	1 small serving (70g)	1 regular serving (84g)
White rice	⅓ serving (46g)	½ serving (66g)
Couscous	⅓ serving (46g)	½ serving (66g)
Sweetcorn	½ cob (60g)	1 small cob (88g)
Boiled potato	2 small (74g)	3 small (106g)
Baked potato	1 medium (59g)	1 large (84g)
French fries	6–7 chips (47g)	8–10 chips (68g)
Sweet potato	½ a potato (61g)	1 small potato (88g)

Non-starchy vegetables

You can enjoy these vegetables in almost unlimited quantities because their starch (sugar) content is minimal. Aim to fill half your plate with a selection of:

Alfalfa	Endive	Raw beetroot
Asparagus	Fennel	Raw carrot
Aubergine	Garlic	Rocket
Beansprouts	Kale	Runner beans
Broccoli	Lettuce	Spinach
Brussels sprouts	Mangetouts	Spring onions
Cabbage	Mushrooms	Tenderstem
Cauliflower	Onions	Tomatoes
Celery	Peas	Watercress
Courgette	Peppers	
Cucumber	Radish	

Low-GL breakfasts

The same essential principles apply to breakfast, although you'll be eating different kinds of foods. My three favourite simple low-GL breakfasts are:

1 Oat flakes or porridge (5GL portion) with berries or apple (5GL portion) and chia seeds or almonds (protein).

2 Two scrambled eggs (protein) on a thin slice of rye or pumpernickel bread (10GL carb portion).

3 A serving of Get Up & Go, with 300ml oat milk, a handful of berries and 1 teaspoon of chia seeds (10GLs – balanced for protein and carbs).

In Chapter 4 I give you some more simple breakfast options.

Low-GL snacks

On the fast days you are allowed one snack; on the feast days, up to three (or two if you choose to have 10GLs of starchy carb portions with main meals). Again, snacks need to be balanced to contain both protein and carbohydrate. Here are some examples:

1 A piece of fruit, plus 5 almonds or 1 dessertspoon of pumpkin seeds.

2 A thin piece of bread or 2 oatcakes and ½ small tub of cottage cheese (150g).

3 A thin piece of bread/2 oatcakes and ¼ small tub of hummus (50g).

4 A thin piece of bread/2 oatcakes and peanut butter.

5 Crudités (a carrot, pepper, cucumber or celery) and ¼ small tub of hummus (50g).

6 Crudités and ½ small tub of cottage cheese (150g).

7 A small plain yoghurt (150g), no sugar, plus berries, or a soya berry yoghurt (no sugar).

8 Cottage cheese plus berries.

In Chapter 4 I give you more simple and delicious snack options.

3

Boosting Your Diet with Exercise

I'm Kate Staples, and I'm a tremendous fan of Patrick's Alternate-Day Low-GL Diet. I recommend it to people who come to my fitness camps and find they are impressed by the health and energy improvements as well as instant weight-loss results. Coupled with the right exercise routine, which doesn't have to take much time at all, the diet is a winning formula. On our recent trial at my fitness camp using Patrick's formula, we had numerous clients seeing remarkable results: up to 3–4lb (1.3–1.8kg) a week of fat loss.

The perfect exercise routine is a combination of resistance exercise that tones and strengthens the body and endurance exercise that builds up your aerobic capacity, both burning calories and boosting your metabolism. A balanced combination of strength and cardiovascular (cardio) training is vital for body shape, body function, body durability and greater health inside and out. All of which leads to a positive state of mind, clarity and confidence.

A toned and strengthened body also enjoys effective metabolism, making it far more efficient at burning fuel and defending itself against unwanted fat accumulation. This is because a strong body is one containing toned muscle – and muscle absorbs glucose. If you have little muscle and your blood sugar goes up, more of the blood sugar will be dumped into the liver and turned into fat. Therefore, the more muscle you have, the more fat you can burn. Muscle burns three times more calories than fat, and lean muscle will keep on performing this important job even while you are asleep.

As you age, your muscle declines, unless you concentrate on your fitness. After the age of 40 you lose up to 1 per cent of your muscle mass each year – that's about half a pound (225g) in a year, about 5 pounds (2.25kg) in a decade.

Both men and women build muscle through exercise, although it appears differently on women. The female body becomes toned but not bulky, so don't worry about the possibility of ending up with big, bulging muscles if you are a woman. In fact, resistance, or strength, training makes you look trimmer, not bulkier and, as we have seen earlier, a pound (450g) of muscle occupies a fraction of the space of an equal amount of fat.

You should aim to do the strength training in this book every other day. On the other days, you should aim for the equivalent of a 30-minute session of power walking or other cardio exercise. For best results, you need to do this three days a week, although you could do the cardio on the same days as the 8-

minute resistance workout if you choose. Exactly what you do, and how you do it, will be explained clearly in the next two chapters. Exercises are grouped according to your current level of fitness, and you will also find a video of each exercise routine on the Internet, so you can work out with me leading you in your living room at home.

Exercise hones the body so that it works better and looks great

The human body is a remarkable tool. It is the machine that allows us to function in a vast array of physical tasks we face during a lifetime – from the most simple and basic movements to extreme challenges of power, endurance, mobility, speed and resilience. It is complex and versatile, capable of extraordinary performance and fantastic recovery, from both exertion and injury; however, for optimum strength, stamina, durability and mobility – as well as longevity – it must be looked after and worked on.

Most people are not aiming for high athletic performance but just want to be in good shape to allow them to work, play and undertake daily activities with ease, and without impairment or pain. Most of us like to look good, too, and a fit, healthy body is, by popular consensus, a more attractive proposition than an unhealthy de-conditioned one.

This is why the simple training routine in this book is so essential for ensuring you get the most from the Alternate-Day Low-GL Diet.

Strength training

Resistance, or strength, training tones and strengthens the body, and it is also one of the best fat-burning secrets around. The fastest and most effective way of boosting your metabolism is to (1) build lean muscle and (2) combine strength training with interval training for cardio fitness. (More on this shortly.)

Through strength training you will also benefit from improved posture, and studies also confirm other health benefits, including a reduction in your risk of diabetes, heart disease, stress, high blood pressure and dementia, according to a recent review in the *British Medical Journal*.[20] Keeping adequately fit also strengthens your bones and protects you from osteoporosis later in life. According to sports medicine professor Wayne Derman, from the University of Cape Town, 'Exercise is the closest thing to an anti-ageing pill.' Recent research indicates that it may add years to the lifespan of your body cells by a process that that protects the DNA by lengthening a component called telomeres, the blueprint for making healthy cells.[21]

What exactly is resistance training?

Resistance training is when you exercise your body against resistance – such as lifting weights – and this builds up the muscle. There are many tools that you can use to do my simple strength-training workout routines, from using drinks bottles as weights to using dumbbells (free weights). Dumbbells are cheap and easy to get hold of (see Resources). There's also the most effective and practical resistance tool of all: using your own bodyweight, such as in a push-up.

Resistance training is suitable for everyone

On my fitness camps I meet people who worry that they won't get fit because they can't run. I tell them that this is not important because it will be the *resistance* work that gets them into shape. I have worked with hundreds of clients who have lost up to 12 inches (30cm) in just one month, and they have enjoyed the process too!

Once you start training and eating well, you will very quickly notice mental changes, and within just three weeks you will start to notice a difference in your body too.

My preferred exercises are known as compound exercises, because they employ different muscle groups simultaneously and involve movement around two or more joints. These kinds of exercises more accurately replicate normal body movement required on a daily basis, such as pushing, pulling and lifting.

Cardio exercises are also a vital part of your exercise regime, so you will be getting the best of all possible worlds in the shortest amount of time. The routines are intended to be practised little and often, making them manageable, practical and easy to build into your life.

Cardio training

The heart is the body's engine, and it's also a muscle that needs to be worked on – and worked out – in the same way as the muscles in the rest of the body. Training that gets your cardio-vascular system – your heart and blood circulation – working efficiently is called cardio training, or aerobic activity. It makes your heart rate go up, along with your breathing, to get into what is called the 'aerobic' zone.

A healthy heart is much less likely to suffer disease than one that is not exercised, and aerobic exercise also promotes healthy blood circulation, which defends the body against debilitating and potentially fatal conditions such as strokes.

A disturbing fact is that three times more women are currently dying of heart disease than of breast cancer, and the risk of heart disease in the UK for a woman over the age of 50 is much the same as for men of the same age, whereas younger women have a lesser risk than men. Heart care is of primary importance to everyone. Regular aerobic workouts are essential if you want to live a long, healthy and active life. They lower cholesterol and reduce blood pressure, as well as delivering a fantastic level of sustained energy.

My alternate-day Exercise Workout will lead you through 30 minutes of cardio training three or four times a week. The selection of activities include:

Walking

Jogging

Biking

Hiking

Swimming

Running stairs

Skipping

Racket sports

Race walking

Cross-country skiing

Dancing

Rowing

Kickboxing

Enjoy yourself

You need to choose activities that you will enjoy, so that you'll get the most pleasure and be more likely to stick to an exercise routine. I'm not an advocate of working yourself into the ground and ending up on the floor feeling sick, which is why the routines are aimed at effective exercise without pushing yourself to extremes. It is important that you enjoy making your sessions a part of your daily routine and that you value them and look forward to them.

Interval training – my favourite 30-minute cardio workout

You may already have heard about interval training. It's the quickest route towards shaping up, because it really fires up your metabolism. It's called interval training because it is a way of mixing intervals of higher- and lower-intensity workouts. It is highly versatile and adaptable, which is why it is used throughout the highest echelons of elite sport, but it is also something an exercise novice can quickly benefit from.

In your 30-minute interval training session as a beginner, you will alternate spurts of lower-intensity walking for 2 minutes with higher intensity walking for 2 minutes. For a more advanced cardio session, alternate your spurts of 2 minutes' walking with 2 minutes of jogging, or to push yourself even further start adding jogging up hills or do 2 minutes of jogging and 2 minutes of harder running. You can even do these sessions on a treadmill at the gym if it is more convenient or when the weather is too unpleasant to be outside.

One of your cardio training sessions per week should be as interval training, depending on your level of fitness. The other cardio sessions can be whatever you choose from the list on page 41.

After your cardio session, cool down by stretching out your leg muscles (see page 75–6). Warm-ups and cool-downs are important, because they help you to avoid injury.

Exercise is not a pastime, a hobby or a luxury – it is a necessity. And as we get older it becomes increasingly necessary. With age, the body can slow down, become more limited, less functional and more prone to put on weight, in particular abdominal fat – but only if left unchecked. The good news is that it is not only possible to keep ageing in check but we can also actually reverse the process. We really can stop the clock and rewind. We don't stop being active because we age: we age because we stop being active.

The Alternate-Day Low-GL Diet and Exercise Workout is based on years of study, research and successful practical application across thousands of people. It will elevate your metabolic rate, create lean muscle, boost energy and vitality, and destroy fat. The workout will kick your metabolism into high gear and keep it there, turning your body into a high-performance fat-burning machine.

You don't need to accept podgy midsections, flabby arms and cellulite. I will show you how to eliminate them and enjoy the life-enhancing and energising process of doing so.

4

The Diet and Exercise Workout in Practice

The secret of burning fat fast is to combine three essential principles in one simple routine:

- Eat an average of 45GLs a day to keep insulin levels down.

- Create a 30 per cent difference in GLs between the moderate fast days (35GLs) and the feast days (50GLs) and a maximum of 800 calories on the fast days.

- Practise the perfect combination of cardio and strength training.

The recipes that follow take all this into account, so you won't have to do any calorie or GL counting; however, you can also freewheel and work out your own 10GL main meals using the charts in Chapter 2.

The key is to have three alternate days a week sticking strictly to 35GLs, which means three 10GL main meals and one 5GL snack. A typical weekly routine would look like this:

Diet	Exercise
MONDAY low-GL 35/below 800 calories	30-minute cardio workout
TUESDAY low-GL 50	8-minute strength workout
WEDNESDAY low-GL 35/below 800 calories	30-minute cardio workout
THURSDAY low-GL 50	8-minute strength workout
FRIDAY low-GL 35/below 800 calories	30-minute cardio workout
SATURDAY day off	day off
SUNDAY low-GL 50	8-minute strength workout

You'll notice in the list above that there is one day when you don't follow the diet or the exercise routine, and for the other days you will be eating an average of about 45GLs per day spread over the week. Many people choose not to have a day off, but it's there as a 'buffer' if you want it. If you blow the diet one day and go off the low-GL track, just count that as your day off. Even if you do have a day off, it's good to make reasonably sensible choices, staying away from sugary foods and eating tons of carbohydrates such as bread, biscuits, pastries, sweets and sweetened drinks.

Similarly, with the exercises, your main goal is to have three strength workouts and three cardio workouts in a week. When you do them it is up to you – and because you won't be using very heavy weights for your strength workouts you don't need to factor in a day's rest between strength workouts to allow your body to repair and build muscle.

If you're familiar with my low-GL diet, you'll know that this also recommends a daily average of 45GLs, so the total amount of food you'll eat in a week isn't different. What *is* different is having alternate feast and moderate fast days, which, as I have discussed earlier, will bring much faster results. Here's how to do it.

What and when to eat on fast days

The goal here is to eat 35GLs in the day and not exceed 800 calories. (Don't worry so much about counting the calories – all the recipes given are in the right ballpark, averaging 250 calories and allowing room for one snack.) The simplest way to do this is to have three 10GL meals a day and one 5GL snack. My advice is to delay eating for at least an hour on waking, and to leave at least two hours between dinner and going to sleep. Do, however, eat in the evening, because it is harder to go to sleep if your blood sugar level is low (or very high).

Eat any *three* of the following suggestions, all designed to keep your blood sugar even with a low GL. The GLs and calories are given for each suggestion and, although listed in the order of breakfasts and main meals, it doesn't matter what you choose and when you eat it. Some people, for example, have the shake, Get Up & Go, twice a day on fasting days, and one other meal. Others have a breakfast option, then soup twice a day. As long as you choose THREE of the MEAL options below you'll be on track. Also, choose ONE of the SNACK options.

You will notice that many of the food recommendations are based on vegetarian protein sources such as beans, lentils and chickpeas. This is because plant-based proteins tend to be significantly lower in calories than animal proteins. This means when you choose a vegetarian option, you get more for your 800 calories. I have also included a good selection of fish choices to ensure you have a good intake of valuable omega-3 fats. What is more, dairy products, and to a lesser extent meat, tend to raise IGF-1, which is counterproductive to switching on the 'skinny' genes.

All the recipes combine protein with carbohydrate, which lowers the GL of the meal. Here are some other ways to further lower the GL of a meal.

- Include foods with high levels of soluble fibre, found in oats and chia seeds, as well as aubergine and okra.

- Another way to increase soluble fibre and fill you up is to take 1 teaspoon, or three capsules, of CarboSlow (glucomannan fibre) or PGX with a large glass of water (see Resources).

- Sip water with a meal, or have a soup, because this fills the stomach and makes you less hungry.

- Add a squeeze of lemon or lime (citric acid) to a meal to slow down gastric emptying, which lowers the GL. So too does adding vinegar to a salad, or having a drizzle of balsamic vinegar on your vegetables.

Breakfasts

- Get Up & Go shake (see Resources) made with 250ml soya milk or skimmed milk and 250ml water and a handful of berries. This is fewer than 300 calories, so you can enjoy this twice on your fasting days, in the morning and afternoon, with a fruit snack or salad in between. Add 1 tsp chia seeds for protein, omega-3s and fibre. To fill you up and lower GL, take 1 tsp, or three capsules, of CarboSlow (glucomannan fibre) or PGX with a glass of water (see Resources). (290 calories)

- A bowl of porridge, made from a small cupful of oats and cooked with 150ml water, 75ml milk plus 3 tsp of chia seeds and berries. An alternative to the berries is ½ chopped or stewed apple, with some cinnamon. (245 calories)

- Yoghurt and berries – a handful of blueberries topped with 100g of natural sheep's, goat's or soya yoghurt sprinkled with 6 chopped or flaked almonds. (210 calories)

- 2 eggs scrambled, boiled or poached – with 2 rough oatcakes or a thin slice of rye or pumpernickel bread. Plus an optional 25g slice of salmon. (270 calories + 40 if adding salmon)

- Spiced apple – gently stew 1 chopped apple with a little water and ground cinnamon to taste. Cool and serve with Greek or soya natural yoghurt and a sprinkle of walnuts. (210 calories)

- Low-GL granola, made with 50g oats, 50g Lizi's Low-GL Granola (available in supermarkets in the UK and by mail order – see Resources) plus a handful of berries to sweeten, and oat, soya or skimmed milk plus 3 tsp chia or pumpkin seeds. If you can't get a low-GL granola, just use another 50g oats instead. (300 calories)

- Scottish kipper fillet with 1 slice of wholemeal toast. The kipper provides a good source of essential omega-3 fats and will keep you feeling full for a good 3–4 hours. (310 calories)

Salads

A substantial serving of any of these salads makes 10GLs. Or have half a portion for a 5GL snack.

- Apple and Tuna Salad (see recipe on page 78) – tuna is a great source of brain-friendly essential fats as well as other vital nutrients and protein. Combining it with apple is a little unusual, but it's very tasty. (168 calories per serving)

- Butternut Squash Salad – toss a handful of thinly sliced oven-baked squash with steamed spears of broccoli, mixed salad leaves and 6 chopped sun-dried tomatoes and 1 slice of grilled halloumi cheese. Dress the salad with vinaigrette. Serve warm or cold. (270 calories)

- Walnut and Three-Bean Salad (see recipe on page 78–9) – no foods are better than beans for satisfying your appetite and giving you stamina. It helps if they're served in a delicious, crunchy salad such as this one. (310 calories per serving)

- Salmon-Stuffed Avocado – scoop the flesh from two halves of a small avocado, mash with 3 tbsp smoked salmon pieces plus lemon juice and black pepper to taste. Spoon back into the skins and serve with a mixed green salad. (215 calories)

- Peruvian Quinoa Salad – mix 85g cooked quinoa, with chopped fresh coriander and parsley, chopped spring onions, ½ garlic clove, 6 cherry tomatoes, some sliced cucumber and ¼ avocado, plus 3 tsp pumpkin seeds and a drizzle of olive oil. Season and serve. (235 calories)

- Feta Salad – to a handful of mixed salad leaves add 6 halved Kalamata olives, 2 chopped sun-dried tomatoes and 2 chopped fresh tomatoes, 25g cubed feta cheese, plus 3 tsp pine nuts and a sprinkle of dried oregano. (240 calories)

- Quinoa Tabbouleh (see recipe on page 79–80) – using quinoa instead of bulgur wheat for this traditional Middle Eastern dish provides first-class protein. Double up the quantities and keep some in the fridge to take to work, if you like. (273 calories per serving)

Soups

Eat a big bowl of vegetable or bean-based soup, which gives you a 300–350g serving (see recipes on pages 80–5), and serve with 2 rough oatcakes (about 45 calories each)

- Beany Vegetable Soup (see recipe on pages 81–1) – this one-pot winter warmer is crammed full of fibre and is useful to take in a vacuum flask to work. (193 calories)

- Chestnut and Butterbean Soup (see recipe on page 81) – chestnuts have the lowest fat content of all nuts and a pleasantly sweet flavour that goes well with the smooth texture of the butter beans. (176 calories)

- Lentil and Lemon Soup (see recipe on pages 81–2) – the spices and lemony sharpness make this lentil soup anything but boring. It's a satisfying winter warmer. (140 calories)

- Spicy Pumpkin and Tofu Soup (see recipe on pages 82–3) – a tasty soup that is a completely balanced meal, with hidden protein power from the tofu. (161 calories)

- High-Energy Lentil Soup (see recipe on pages 83–4) – this soup is packed with vitamin A from the carrots and tomatoes, as well as health-giving garlic, making it especially good for those times when you are feeling tired and stressed, which makes you vulnerable to infections. (197 calories)

- Quick Pea and Mint Soup (see recipe on pages 84–5) – although very simple to make, this fresh-tasting soup looks and tastes good enough to serve for a dinner party. (243 calories)

Other main meals

- Pasta with Borlotti Bolognese (see recipe on pages 85–6) – here's a simple sauce recipe with three low-GL pasta variations to try: courgette 'pasta', chickpeas or wholemeal pasta. (217 calories)

- Indian Spiced Chicken – marinate 1 chicken breast in a blend of the juice of 1 lemon, 1 crushed garlic clove, ½ tsp each of ground turmeric and cumin, 1 tsp ground coriander and a pinch of cayenne for at least 30 minutes. Grill for 15 minutes turning halfway through the cooking time. Serve with a large portion of greens such as Tenderstem broccoli, or a salad. (195 calories per serving)

- Roasted Cod – mix ½ tbsp each of olive oil and chopped fresh parsley and 1 crushed garlic clove. Rub over a portion of cod (or haddock or plaice) fillet and leave for 10 minutes, then oven bake at 180°C/350°F/Gas 4 for 10 minutes. Serve with a tomato and onion salad and 100g cooked brown rice, couscous or two boiled potatoes. (109 calories + 150 calories for the brown rice, couscous or boiled potatoes)

- Steamed Salmon – steam a portion of salmon gently for 10–14 minutes in a steamer over a pan of boiling water. (Try to go for wild salmon, as it's a healthier option than farmed fish.) Serve on a bed of thinly sliced cooked greens stir-fried with garlic and soy sauce and topped with stir-fried sliced spring onions. Serve with 100g cooked brown rice or 200g cooked quinoa. (110 calories for salmon + 150 calories for rice or 85 calories for quinoa)

- Three-Egg Omelette – the best kind of fast food. Add a thin slice of smoked salmon plus 2 asparagus spears (295 calories), or wilted spinach and sun-dried tomato (300 calories), or stir-fried shiitake mushrooms (240 calories) as a filling.

- Chickpea and Spinach Curry (see recipe on pages 86–7) – this delicious low-GL curry is perfect for vegetarian food lovers. (216 calories + 85 calories for quinoa)

- Garlic Chilli Prawns with Pak Choi (see recipe on pages 87–8) – this prawn dish is delicious and quick to cook. (250 calories + 85 calories for quinoa)

- Salmon Fillets with New Potatoes (see recipe on pages 88–9) – salmon not only provides plenty of protein but is also a source of essential fats. Vegetarians could marinate tofu slices instead of using salmon. (225 calories, 165 if using tofu, plus 70 calories for 3 baby new potatoes)

- Trout with Puy Lentils and Roasted Tomatoes on the Vine (see recipe on pages 89–90) – a simple but sophisticated dish that is perfectly balanced and smart enough to serve at a dinner party. (285 calories)

Snacks

Each of these snacks is 5GLs. On fast days have one snack; on feast days have two or three if you want to, but you don't have to. Many people find they are just not that hungry.

- A small apple, pear or peach (about 60 calories), plus five almonds (35 calories) or a tablespoon of pumpkin seeds (60 calories). Half an apple and almonds is 65 calories.

- A small, natural bio yoghurt (150g), no sugar, plus a handful of berries (100 calories).

- One thin slice of Scandinavian-style rye or pumpernickel bread with a thin spread of sugar-free peanut butter (100 calories).

- Lean meat or fish, such as smoked salmon (no more than 100g), with a thin slice of Scandinavian-style rye bread or one or two rough Nairn's oatcakes – double the portion for a main meal. (Snack 120–150 calories, or 80–100 calories with one oatcake)

- A 50g serving of one of the following dips, with either vegetable sticks (carrot, cucumber, peppers) or an oatcake:

  Mexican Bean Dip (see recipe on page 90). (47 calories)
  Homemade Hummus (see recipe on page 91). (112 calories)
  Baba Ganoush (see recipe on pages 91–2). (75 calories)
  Smoked Salmon Pâté (see recipe on page 92). (97 calories)
  Cottage cheese (½ small tub, 150g). (67 calories)

- Spiced Chickpeas (see recipe on pages 92–3) – a low-fat, savoury snack rich in combined protein and low-GL carbs, 100g serving. (105 calories)

- Gazpacho Andaluz (see recipe on pages 93–4) – for a taste of Andalusia, serve this raw cold soup at alfresco meals or for a perfect instant snack. It stores well in the fridge for up to one week. Add black-eyed beans to make it a main meal – and an ice cube or two on really sultry days, 140g serving. (102 calories)

- Creamy Coleslaw (see recipe on page 94) – cabbage, carrots and onions are rich in vitamins and minerals, and this home-made coleslaw tastes much better than the supermarket variety, 50g serving. (103 calories)

What to eat on feast days

On the feast days, follow my low-GL diet, as explained in Chapter 2. You can also read more about the diet in my books *The Low-GL Diet Bible*, *The Low-GL Diet Made Easy* and *The*

Low-GL Diet Cookbook. The recipes in these books allow for 45GLs per day, including two 5GL snacks and 5GLs for a drink or dessert; on your feast days you'll be allowed 10GLs more carbohydrate.

Base your meals on the plate explained on pages 29–30; that is with one-quarter as protein, one-quarter as starchy carbohydrate and half as non-starchy vegetable carbohydrate. Eating in this way is calculated on the basis of 3GLs for the vegetable portion and 7GLs for the starchy carb portion.

Your allowance on a feast day is a bit more than my standard low-GL diet of 45GLs, giving you 50GLs in a day, so you can be more lenient and have a 10GL portion of starchy carbohydrate in a meal (see pages 31–2). In the books listed above you will find these variations listed as 'maintenance' portions, because these are the higher levels of carbohydrate you can eat when you have achieved your target weight. Alternatively, you could have one more 5GL snack, or a double portion of a snack.

The main-meal suggestions for the feast days still apply, although you don't have to be so strict on the carb portion, using the chart on page 32 as a guide.

The snack suggestions, being 5GLs, also apply, but you can have two 5GL snacks a day if you are eating 'maintenance' portion sizes for main meals, and three a day if you are not. Some people who wake up early to exercise, for example, have a low-GL snack on rising, perhaps before exercising, then have breakfast an hour or so later. In the books listed above you'll find lots of snack suggestions, plus small-meal ideas and recipes.

The best drinks

On both fast and feast days the best drinks of all are water and teas (herbal, green or weak black), which have no GLs. It is better to avoid strong coffee, or have a maximum of one a day, and avoid other caffeinated drinks. The combination of coffee and carbohydrate snacks raises both blood sugar and insulin levels very high, promoting insulin resistance.

Make sure you drink plenty of water when you are exercising. It is best to start training hydrated, so drink 250ml water at least 30 minutes before training. During training take regular sips but not an excessive amount of fluids. You need about a 1.5 litres of water on a day when you are exercising.

When to exercise and eat

The body repairs and rebuilds muscle better when supplied with a combination of low-GL carbs and protein, which are contained in all the meal options. I recommend you exercise before one of your meals, and eat within 30 minutes of completing your workout – either a low-GL snack or a main meal.

You can also choose to have your low-GL snack before your cardio exercise to give you some energy.

You could exercise in the morning, before breakfast, or in the early evening, before dinner. But don't exercise too late, as you should start relaxing in the evening for a good night's sleep.

The exercise routines are fully described in Chapter 5.

Recommended supplements

I recommend you supplement chromium, HCA (from tamarind) and 5-HTP (a form of tryptophan). These supplements support normal blood sugar and insulin regulation. Some supplements contain all three of the above, where you take one capsule/tablet just before each meal. (Please note that 5-HTP is not recommended if you are on antidepressant drugs.) An alternative is chromium with a cinnamon extract.

I always recommend supplementing a high-potency multivitamin–mineral, 1g of vitamin C and essential omegas (both omega-3 from fish oil and omega-6 from borage or evening primrose oil) twice a day. These are not only good for general health but also support metabolism and satisfy the body's need for nutrients, hence reducing food cravings. If you take in enough essential fats you'll have fewer cravings for fat. Omega-3 fats, from supplements or oily fish, also turn off inflammation and may help turn on some of these positive anti-ageing genes.

There is no need to supplement a multivitamin–mineral and 1g of vitamin C when you have the Get Up & Go shake, because this already includes sufficient vitamins and minerals. If you have a serving of oily fish on that day you are also covered for omega-3 fats.

Another optional extra to switch on the 'skinny' sirtuin genes, is resveratrol. There's a debate about how much to take, ranging from 20 to 5,000mg a day. In animal studies, doses of around 300mg (the human equivalent) seem to trigger genetic expression similar to calorie restriction.[22] High-potency resveratrol is available as a supplement (see Resources).

What to do when you have reached your goal

Feedback from volunteers on regular fasting diets shows that people are reaching their goals more quickly than on regular diets and that alternate-day fasting has turbo-charged their progress. I expect you to achieve your goals more quickly on the Alternate-Day Low-GL Diet and Exercise Workout, because you will be benefiting from alternate-day fasting *and* a low-GL diet *and* structured exercise. So what should you do when you get there? In order to exploit the longer-term benefits of CR and intermittent fasting, I suggest you follow this pattern:

- One day: the modified fast, following the same rules as above – that is a maximum of 35GLs and 800 calories.

- Six days: follow the low-GL principles using 45–60GLs. You will discover what level of GLs supports maintenance of your weight and gives you the most health benefits. For some people, this may be 55GLs, whereas for others it may be 40 or 45GLs. You will need to experiment a little to find what works best for you.

You will want to continue with your fitness routine even after you have met your goals, because by now you will be enjoying it and probably can't imagine life without exercise.

5

The Alternate-Day Workout Routines

I n this chapter you will find instructions for the cardio and strength-training workouts. There are three levels for the strength training – beginner, intermediate and advanced – and you will find that the exercises are divided into these three groups. Each exercise is illustrated, and you can also watch an online video demonstrating the routines, so you will easily learn the exercises that make up your 8-minute strength-training programme. As you become fitter you can progress through the levels. You'll find the video at www.zest4life.com/burnfatfastexercises.

Remember that every other day you'll be doing a cardio workout consisting of 30 minutes. You can choose of any of these activities:

Walking

Jogging

Biking

Hiking

Swimming

Running stairs

Skipping

Racket sports

Race walking

Cross-country skiing

Dancing

Rowing

Kickboxing

Interval training (2 minutes

jogging/running plus 2 minutes

walking, for 30 minutes)

During your cardio workout, you are aiming to increase your heart rate by up to 50 per cent, so if your resting heart rate is normally 80 beats per minute you are aiming to push it up to about 120 beats. You can work with your breath while exercising to gauge this level. Exhale on the exertion, and you should be sweating a little at a level where you are just about able to talk. Your target is three cardio workouts a week.

In addition, you need to do three strength workouts a week. Each session begins with a warm-up, then the sequence will take 8 minutes for beginners and slightly longer for the more advanced programme. The most important thing is to listen to your body while exercising so that you know when you need to take a rest or slow down. Each workout consists of four exercises. The chart below shows you the exercises at a glance. See below for the number of repetitions, and any equipment you will need.

To determine which category of programme you should start with, here is a guideline. If in doubt, start with the beginner's workout and progress when you feel ready.

Beginner For those returning to exercise post-injury or if you are not used to any regular activity.

Intermediate For those currently exercising for approximately 2–3 hours a week.

Advanced For those currently exercising for approximately 3 hours-plus a week.

Beginner	Intermediate	Advanced
Wall Sit	Squat Shoulder Press	Jumping Squats
Modified Box Press	Box Press with Alternate Leg Lift	Full Press-up
Plank Step-outs	Plank Jacks	Mountain Climbers
Alternate Reverse Lunge	Reverse Lunge with Triceps Kick Back	Pendulum Lunge

Time and required equipment

Beginner Each exercise takes 45 seconds. Do the entire sequence twice. You will need a mat and a water bottle.

Intermediate Each exercise takes 60 seconds. Do the entire sequence twice. You will need a mat and dumbbells (women 2kg; men 3–4kg).

Advanced Each exercise takes 60 seconds. Do the entire sequence three times. You will need a mat and dumbbells (women 2–5kg; men 4–6kg).

Do as many repetitions of the exercises within each 45/60 minute set as you can do comfortably. As you get fitter you'll do more.

Warm-up

First, you need to increase your heart rate to prepare your body to perform the tasks ahead, so that you will avoid any strains or injury. This isn't complicated and this should be an enjoyable experience and something that you can fit into your daily schedule with ease. Warm-ups include hill walking, slow jogging, walking up and down the stairs, dancing and using a stationary bike. Just do something that gets your heart pumping. This should take you about 5 minutes.

If you want to combine your cardio workout with your strength workout, start with the warm-up, then do some strength training and progress to the cardio workout.

As long as you have three cardio workouts and three strength workouts a week, how you achieve those goals is up to you.

Your strength workout

As outlined in Chapter 3, strength training is the heart and soul of fitness and has many benefits, helping you to burn more calories than you can through cardio over a 24-hour period. And it will help to switch on those 'skinny' genes.

The exercises focus on the main muscles used for strengthening, toning and adding definition, including the chest, upper and lower back, abdominal/core muscles (or abs), and the four major muscle groups in your legs, your buttocks, glutes (bottom), quadriceps, also called quads (front thigh), hamstrings (back thigh) and the triceps (the back of your arms).

Beginner's programme

WALL SIT

Targets your bottom/glutes, inner thigh, quads and hamstrings.
45 seconds × 2 sets

How to do it:

1 Squat against the wall, cross your arms and look straight ahead
  with your back flat and pressed against the wall.
2 Your legs ideally need to be at 90 degrees to the wall, no more.
3 Feet in line with your knees.
4 Push with your quads into the wall.

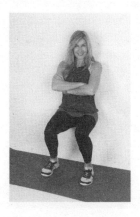

MODIFIED BOX PRESS

Targets your chest, back and abdominal/core muscles.
45 seconds × 2 sets

How to do it:

1 Kneel on all fours with your hands shoulder-width apart and under
  your shoulders; knees and toes on the floor.
2 With your elbows bent, drop your chest towards the floor that so
  you are nearly touching the floor. Straighten your elbows as you
  push back up to your starting position. Build up to 45 seconds;
  stop when you experience muscle fatigue.
3 Pay attention to the following points:
  • Focus on engaging your chest muscles as you push off the mat.
  • Keep your abdominals engaged and your hips level.
  • Use controlled movements, breathing out on the way up.
  • Don't lock out your elbows.
  • Don't arch your back.

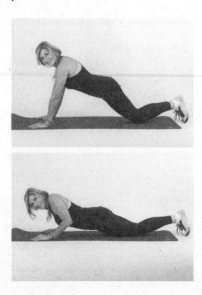

PLANK STEP-OUTS

Targets your core and shoulders.
45 seconds × 2 sets

How to do it:

1 Position yourself on your front in a full push-up position with your body in a straight line from head to toe and your hands shoulder-width apart and directly underneath your shoulders, arms straight. You are supporting your weight on your hands and toes.
2 With a straight leg, step out to the right and tap the outside of the mat, if using one, or at about 10 inches (25cm) away from the leg's start position, then bring it back to the centre.
3 Repeat with the other leg and continue for 45 seconds.
4 Pay attention to the following points:
   • Keep your abs engaged and avoid arching your back.
   • Keep your eyes focused on the floor with your head in line with your body.

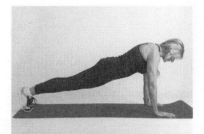

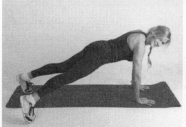
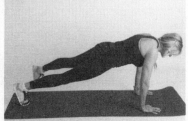

ALTERNATE REVERSE LUNGE

Targets your quads, hamstrings and glutes.
45 seconds × 2 sets

How to do it:

1 Stand upright with your hands on your hips and your feet
  shoulder-width apart.
2 Take a step backwards, dropping your back knee to a few inches
  above the floor without touching the floor.
3 Your knees should be in line with your toes and both legs bent into
  a 90-degree angle.
4 Your weight should be on the front leg.
5 Push off with your front foot to return to the start position.
6 Step back with the other leg and repeat the sequence.

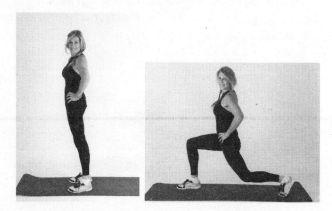

Remember: all the exercises can be seen at
www.zest4life.com/burnfatfastexercises

Intermediate programme

SQUAT SHOULDER PRESS

Targets your quads, hamstrings, glutes, core, lower back and shoulders.
60 seconds × 2 sets

How to do it:

1 Stand with feet shoulder-width apart, holding dumbbells by your shoulders.
2 Squat down, with your back straight, and push your glutes (bottom) back.
3 Stand up by pressing your feet into the floor before your legs are fully straight.
4 Press the dumbbells straight up, while trying to keep your arms in line with your ears.

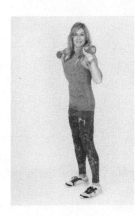 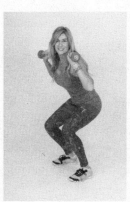 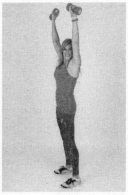

Box Press with Alternate Leg Lift

Targets your chest, upper back, shoulders and core.
60 seconds × 2 sets or 20 reps each leg

How to do it:

1 Kneel on all fours with your hands shoulder-width apart and directly under your shoulders; knees on the floor.
2 Lower your chest towards the mat.
3 Push up and, as you come off the floor, lift one knee 6 inches (5cm) off the floor. Drop your chest to the floor and repeat with the other leg.
4 Alternate this movement with every push-up.

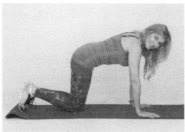

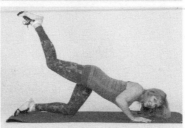

Plank Jacks

Challenge your cardio with this exercise. It targets your core, shoulders and glutes.
60 seconds × 2 sets

How to do it:

1 Position yourself on your front in a push-up position with your body in a straight line from head to toe and your hands shoulder-width apart and directly underneath your shoulders, arms straight. You are supporting your weight on your hands and toes.
2 Jump your feet outwards so that they are outside the mat, if using one, or 12 inches (30cm) from the leg's start position. Now jump back to the centre and repeat.
3 Pay attention to the following points:
   • Keep your back as flat as possible.
   • Don't shift your weight forward or backward with each jump, and try to remain steady with your abs engaged.
   • Keep your shoulders strong, and focus on trying to push the ground away from you as you support yourself in the plank position.

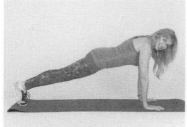 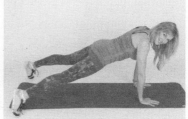

REVERSE LUNGE WITH TRICEPS KICK-BACK

Targets your quads, glutes, triceps and core. Front thigh, bottom, backs of arms and abs/core
60 seconds × 2 sets

How to do it:

1 Stand upright with your hands by your sides, holding your dumbbells.
2 Take a step backwards, dropping your back knee to a few inches above the floor without touching the floor.
3 Keep your elbows squeezed into your sides.
4 Straighten the arms by pushing the dumbbells away from you.
5 Push off with your front foot to return to the start position.
6 Step back with the other leg and repeat the sequence.

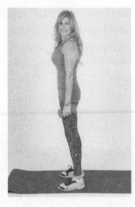 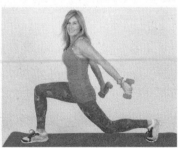

Remember: all the exercises can be seen at www.zest4life.com/burnfatfastexercises

Advanced Programme

JUMPING SQUATS

Fire up your cardio with this exercise, which targets your quads, hamstrings, calves, core and lower back.
60 seconds × 3 sets or 20 jumps each set

How to do it:

1 Stand upright with your hands on your hips.
2 Bend at the hips and knees into a half-squat position, leaning your torso slightly forward and with your arms straight behind you.
3 Push off from your feet, jumping straight up.
4 Land in a semi-squat position and repeat the jump.
5 Land with bent knees to absorb the impact.

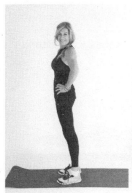
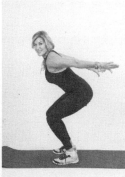
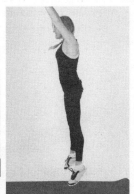

FULL PUSH-UP

Targets your back, shoulders and core.
60 seconds × 3 sets or 20 in each set

How to do it:

1 Position yourself on your front in a full push-up position with your body in a straight line from head to toe and your hands slightly more than shoulder-width apart, arms straight. You are supporting your weight on your hands and toes. Keep your hands and your abs tight and engaged.
2 Inhale as your drop yourself to the floor, stopping as your elbows reach a 90-degree bend.
3 Inhale on the way down and exhale on the way up. Exhale and push yourself away from the floor.
4 Pay attention to the following points:
   • Don't touch the floor on the way down.
   • Don't bend your back.
5 You can modify the exercise by dropping your knees, if necessary.

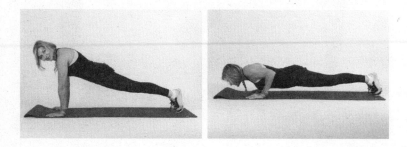

Mountain Climbers

This hard-core cardio exercise targets back, shoulders and core.
60 seconds × 3 sets

How to do it:

1 Position yourself on your front in a full push-up position with your body in a straight line from head to toe and your hands shoulder-width apart and directly underneath your shoulders, arms straight. You are supporting your weight on your hands and toes. Keep your hands and your abs tight and engaged.
2 Support your body on your hands and toes and bring one knee up and draw it into your chest. The other leg is straight out and behind.
3 Alternately jump your feet in and out, bringing your knees into your chest each time.
4 Pay attention to the following point:
   • Keep your fingers spread out and your hands directly under your shoulders throughout.

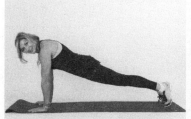 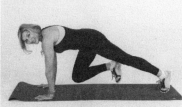

PENDULUM LUNGE

This forward-and-reverse lunge targets the whole of the lower body; all the muscle groups are engaged.
30 seconds each leg × 3 sets

How to do it:

1 Stand upright with your hands on your hips and your feet shoulder-width apart. Lift your right foot off the floor and lunge or step forward to a 90-degree angle, dropping your back knee.
2 Pushing off with the front foot, lift the right foot and drop the knee behind you. Remain on the same leg for 30 seconds and repeat on the other side.
3 Pay attention to the following points:
   • Keep your torso straight and make sure your knee is in line with your toes.
   • Don't tip forward with your body.
   • Keep your chest proud.

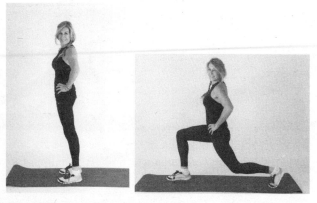

Remember: all the exercises can be seen at
www.zest4life.com/burnfatfastexercises

Cool-down

The cool-down is as important as the warm-up, so that you stretch out your calf stretches, hamstrings and quads. Below you'll find a few of my favourite cool-down stretches. Stretching after exercise will help to avoid any potential injuries and will allow the muscles to lengthen to avoid soreness the following day. Just remember the number one rule of stretching – never bounce on a stretch. Also, do not stretch beyond the point where you begin to feel tightness in the muscle, and never stretch to the point of discomfort or pain.

At the end of your sessions do the following stretches.

CALF STRETCHES

Stand about 3 feet (90cm) from a wall, feet at shoulder width and flat on the ground. Put your hands on the wall with your arms straight for support. Lean your hips forward and bend your knees slightly to stretch your calves.

HAMSTRING STRETCHES

Stand with one leg just in front of the other and bend the back knee. Rest your weight on the bent knee with the hand above the knee joint. Tilt the hips forwards as if sticking your bottom in the air and hold for 10–20 seconds.

QUAD STRETCH

Stand on one foot, with one hand on a wall for balance. Hold the other foot with the opposite hand and raise the heel of the lifted foot to the buttocks (or as close as comfortably possible), stretching your quadriceps. Keep your body upright throughout. Change legs and repeat. Hold each stretch for 15 seconds.

6

The Alternate-Day Low-GL Recipes

All the recipes given here conform to the rules for main meals for both the moderate fast days and the feast days, namely providing no more than 10GLs per recipe. They are also suitably low in calories, averaging 250 calories.

Most are adapted from my *Low-GL Diet Bible* or *The Low-GL Diet Cookbook*, which provide plenty of extra recipes and instructions on how to live a low-GL life. Some recipes have also come from the Holford Zest4Life groups, which are each led by a qualified nutritional therapist or weight-loss coach. See www.zest4life.com for details of groups near you. In case you don't have a group near you, there is also a 'virtual' group called Six Weeks to Success (see page 110). There are plenty of ways you can get more recipes and support to achieve your goals, but there are enough recipes in this book to get you started.

Main Meals

Salads

APPLE AND TUNA SALAD

4GLs (168 calories per serving)
Serves 2

   175g tuna in brine, drained
   1 apple, chopped
   1 celery stick, sliced
   1 little gem lettuce, torn into bite-sized pieces
   1 tbsp low-fat mayonnaise
   85g live natural yogurt
   2 tsp lemon juice
   sea salt and ground black pepper

Drain the tuna and mix well with the remaining ingredients.

WALNUT AND THREE-BEAN SALAD

3GLs (310 calories per serving)
Serves 2

   400g can mixed beans, such as haricot beans, chickpeas and
       flageolet beans
   1 handful of walnuts, roughly chopped
   ½ apple, cubed
   2 tsp chopped fresh parsley or chives

1 tbsp olive oil
1 tbsp walnut oil (or olive oil)
juice of ½ lemon
1 celery stick, finely chopped
sea salt and ground black pepper
mixed salad leaves, such as baby spinach, rocket and watercress,
    to serve

Combine all the ingredients except the salad leaves and serve with the mixed salad.

QUINOA TABBOULEH

8GLs (273 calories per serving)
Serves 2

140g quinoa
350ml stock made with 1 tsp of vegetable bouillon powder
¼ medium cucumber, sliced lengthways into quarters, then finely
    sliced horizontally
2 large handfuls of cherry tomatoes, chopped to the same size as
    the cucumber
4 spring onions, finely sliced
1 large handful of fresh mint, finely chopped
1 large handful of fresh parsley, finely chopped
1–2 tbsp olive oil
1 tbsp lemon juice
2 tsp balsamic vinegar, or to taste
sea salt and ground black pepper

Bring the quinoa to the boil in a pan with the stock, then cover, reduce the heat and simmer for 10–15 minutes until the liquid is absorbed and the grains are fluffy. Put the quinoa in a bowl and leave to cool to room temperature.

Mix in the chopped vegetables and herbs, then add the oil, lemon juice and vinegar. Season. Taste to check the flavour and adjust accordingly. Chill in the fridge for at least 1 hour to allow the flavours to develop.

Soups

BEANY VEGETABLE SOUP

8GLs (193 calories per serving)
Serves 6

  2 onions, chopped
  3 celery sticks, finely chopped
  3 leeks, sliced
  450g mixed root vegetables, such as carrot, swede and parsnip,
    peeled and chopped into bite-sized chunks
  850ml vegetable stock
  2 × 400g cans mixed pulses (or your choice of beans, such as
    kidney, chickpea, borlotti, butter or flageolet), drained and
    rinsed
  2 tbsp roughly chopped fresh parsley
  sea salt and ground black pepper

Put the onion, celery, leeks, root vegetables, stock and seasoning in a large pan and stir. Cover and bring to the boil, then reduce the heat and simmer for 20 minutes.

Stir in the mixed pulses, then cover and simmer for 5–10 minutes until the vegetables and beans are tender. Add the parsley, then check the seasoning before serving.

CHESTNUT AND BUTTERBEAN SOUP

4GLs (176 calories per serving)
Serves 4

200g vacuum-packed or canned cooked and peeled chestnuts
400g can butter beans, drained and rinsed
1 onion, chopped
1 carrot, chopped
2 thyme sprigs
1.2 litres vegetable bouillon or stock
ground black pepper

Put all the ingredients in a large pan and bring to the boil. Cover and simmer very gently for 35 minutes. Purée the soup in a food processor or blender until smooth.

LENTIL AND LEMON SOUP

2GLs (140 calories per serving)
Serves 4

1 tbsp olive oil
250g onions, chopped
4 garlic cloves, coarsely chopped

250g red lentils, rinsed
1.2 litres chicken or vegetable stock
1 tsp ground cumin
1 tsp ground coriander
juice of ½ lemon
sea salt and ground black pepper

Heat the oil in a pan and add the onions and garlic. Cook over low heat, stirring frequently, for 10 minutes or until soft.

Add the lentils and cook for a further 2 minutes. Add the stock and bring to the boil, then reduce the heat to a simmer for 30–45 minutes until the lentils are almost soft.

In a non-stick frying pan, dry-fry the spices over a high heat for 1–2 minutes until they release their aroma, then add to the soup. Bring the soup back to the boil and add the lemon juice, then simmer for 5 minutes. Season lightly and serve.

SPICY PUMPKIN AND TOFU SOUP

6GLs (116 calories per serving)
Serves 4

1 tbsp olive oil
1 large onion, finely chopped
2 garlic cloves, crushed
2 large butternut squash, deseeded, peeled and diced
1½ tsp cumin
1 tsp ground coriander
¼ tsp chilli powder
½ tsp freshly grated nutmeg

1 tsp fresh thyme, chopped

3 vegetable stock cubes dissolved in 1 litre boiling water

1 packet Cauldron Organic Tofu, drained

2 tbsp chopped fresh parsley and chives

sea salt and ground black pepper

Heat the olive oil in a large pan. Add the chopped onion and garlic, and cook over a low heat until the onion has softened.

Add the diced squash, the cumin, coriander, chilli, nutmeg, thyme and stock. Bring to the boil, then reduce the heat and simmer for 15 minutes. Leave to cool slightly.

Whiz the tofu in a food processor or blender and set aside. Blend the soup and return it to the pan. Whisk in the tofu using a balloon whisk, a tablespoonful at a time, and gently reheat. Season to taste, then add the fresh herbs and serve.

(Recipe courtesy of Cauldron Foods)

HIGH-ENERGY LENTIL SOUP

4GLs (197 calories per serving)
Serves 4

1–2 tbsp olive oil

1 large onion, chopped

1 garlic clove, crushed

2 celery sticks, chopped

1 leek, sliced

1 carrot, chopped

200g can chopped tomatoes

1 tsp dried mixed herbs or 1 handful of fresh parsley, finely chopped

200g brown or green lentils
1 litre vegetable stock
ground black pepper

Heat the oil in a large pan and add a splash of water. Cover and cook the onion, celery, leek and garlic over a medium heat, stirring frequently, for 8 minutes or until soft and transparent.

Add the remaining ingredients and stir thoroughly to combine. Bring to the boil, then simmer, covered, for 30–40 minutes until the lentils and vegetables are tender.

Leave to cool slightly, then transfer half the soup to a food processor or blender and blend until smooth. Return the blended soup to the pan, stir well to combine, then reheat and serve.

QUICK PEA AND MINT SOUP

3GLs (243 calories per serving)
Serves 4

1.5kg frozen peas (or fresh peas, or half and half)
1 large bunch fresh mint, plus extra leaves to garnish
1 litre boiling water
4 tsp low-fat crème fraîche
sea salt and ground black pepper
4 rashers lean bacon, grilled and cut into small pieces, or 65g
    crumbled goat's cheese, to serve (optional)

Put the peas and mint into a large pan and add the water. Bring to the boil, then simmer for 3 minutes.

Strain off most of the liquor and retain it, then blend the peas and mint until you have a smooth purée.

Gradually add some of the liquor back into the pan until you achieve the desired consistency. Return to the pan and gently bring back to the boil. Season to taste.

When ready to serve, swirl 1 tsp crème fraîche into each bowl of soup and add a mint leaf. Serve the soup with the crispy bacon or crumbled goat's cheese over the top.

Other main meals

PASTA WITH BORLOTTI BOLOGNESE

10GLs (217 per serving for Borlotti sauce, 40g wholewheat pasta = 130 calories)
Serves 2

1 tbsp olive oil
1 onion, chopped
2 garlic cloves, crushed
1 tsp mixed dried herbs
115g button mushrooms, sliced
1 tsp vegetable bouillon powder
1 tbsp tomato purée
140g canned tomatoes
400g can borlotti beans, drained and rinsed
sea salt and ground black pepper
40g wholegrain spaghetti or pasta, or 75g of chickpea pasta or
    quinoa, or courgette 'pasta' (see tip), to serve

Heat the oil in a pan and fry the onion, garlic and herbs for 2 minutes, then add the mushrooms and cook until soft. Add the vegetable bouillon powder, tomato purée, tomatoes and beans, then season and simmer for 15 minutes. Serve with pasta, quinoa or courgette 'pasta'.

Tip
Make your own courgette pasta by using a grater to slice a courgette into thin ribbons. Put on a baking tray in an oven preheated to 180°C/350°F/Gas 4 for 5 minutes to warm through.

CHICKPEA AND SPINACH CURRY

10GLs (216 calories per serving + 85 calories for 75g quinoa)
Serves 4

    1 tbsp olive oil or coconut oil
    2 red onions, sliced
    1 mild red chilli, deseeded and finely chopped
    1 tbsp mild or medium curry powder, or Madras spice blend
    150ml hot vegetable stock
    500ml coconut milk
    ¼ head of cauliflower, chopped into small chunks
    2 × 410g cans chickpeas, drained and rinsed
    1 tsp sea salt
    200g baby leaf spinach, chopped
    75g cooked quinoa, or a salad of diced cucumber, tomatoes and
       red onion, to serve

Heat 2 tsp of the oil in a large pan and add the onions. Cook over a low heat for 3–4 minutes until softened. Add the chilli and curry powder and cook for a further 1 minute.

Stir in the stock, coconut milk, cauliflower and chickpeas, then simmer for 15 minutes to reduce the sauce and allow the flavours to combine. Season with salt. Add the spinach, stir and cook gently for 2 minutes or until warmed through. Serve with quinoa or salad.

GARLIC CHILLI PRAWNS WITH PAK CHOI

10GLs (250 calories per serving + 85 calories for 75g quinoa or 150 calories for 45g brown rice)
Serves 2

3 garlic cloves, crushed
juice of 2 limes
1 green chilli, deseeded
1 tsp chilli-infused oil or a large pinch dried chilli flakes
3 tbsp virgin rapeseed oil
300g large, raw prawns, prepared
sea salt
75g cooked quinoa or 45g cooked brown rice, to serve

For the pak choi:
1 tbsp virgin rapeseed oil
250g (9oz) pak choi, stems separated, and both stems and leaves roughly chopped
1 tbsp oyster sauce

Put the garlic in a blender and add the lime, chillies, chilli oil or flakes, a good pinch of salt and the oil. Blend into a purée. Put the prawns into a bowl and add the purée. Leave to marinate for 20 minutes at room temperature.

Heat a griddle or frying pan over a medium-high heat. Cook the prawns for 1½ minutes on each side.

Meanwhile, to make the pak choi, heat the oil in a hot wok or frying pan and add the pak choi stems. Stir-fry or steam-fry (by adding a dash of water and then covering) for 1 minute, then add the leaves and cook for 3 minutes. Remove from the heat and stir in the oyster sauce. Serve with the prawns, quinoa or rice.

SALMON FILLETS WITH NEW POTATOES

10GLs (225 calories per serving + 70 calories for new potatoes)
Serves 2

    juice and zest of ½ orange
    1 tsp clear honey
    1 tsp wholegrain mustard
    2 small skinless and boneless salmon fillets
    steam-fried spinach (see tip) and red or yellow peppers, and 6
        boiled baby new potatoes or 45g cooked brown basmati rice to
        serve

Put the orange juice and zest into a small bowl and whisk in the honey and mustard. Put the salmon into a shallow dish and pour over the orange mixture. Leave to marinate for 30 minutes–1 hour, in the fridge. Meanwhile, preheat the oven to 180°C/350°F/gas mark 4.

Bake the salmon for 20–25 minutes until cooked through. Serve with spinach and peppers, baby new potatoes or rice.

Tip
To steam-fry accompanying vegetables add 1 tsp oil or butter and 1 tbsp water or stock to a pan over medium heat and add the vegetables. Cook until tender.

TROUT WITH PUY LENTILS AND ROASTED TOMATOES ON THE VINE

10Gls (calories 285)
Serves 2

> 85g Puy lentils, rinsed
> 1 tsp vegetable bouillon powder
> 1 tsp mixed dried herbs (such as Herbes de Provence)
> 2 small trout fillets (about 100g each)
> ½ bunch cherry tomatoes on the vine (or 5–6 tomatoes per
>   person)
> 2 slices of lemon
> 1 handful of fresh parsley, chopped
> ground black pepper

Put the lentils in a pan and cover with cold water. Bring to the boil, then simmer for 20 minutes or until the water is mostly absorbed. Add the bouillon powder and mixed herbs when the lentils are soft to the bite. (Don't worry if the lentils seem a little hard – Puy lentils retain their shape and have a satisfyingly chewy texture when cooked.)

Meanwhile, preheat the oven to 190°C/375°F/gas mark 5.

Put the fish in a non-stick roasting tin and lay the tomatoes around them, then bake for 12–15 minutes until cooked through.

Put a dollop of lentils onto each plate and lay the fish on top. Add a slice of lemon and chopped parsley to each fillet and put the tomatoes on the side. Sprinkle with black pepper and serve.

MEXICAN BEAN DIP

4GLs (90 calories per serving)
Serves 4

½ tbsp olive oil
¼ onion, finely chopped
2 garlic cloves, crushed
1 tsp chilli powder
140g canned kidney beans, drained and rinsed
1 tsp lemon juice
85g cottage cheese
1 tbsp yogurt
sea salt and ground black pepper

Heat the oil in a pan and fry the onion and garlic gently for 2 minutes, then add the chilli powder and cook for a further 3 minutes. Cool. Blend all the ingredients to make a fairly smooth, creamy dip.

HOMEMADE HUMMUS

5GLs (155 calories per serving)
Serves 4

    400g can chickpeas, drained and rinsed
    2 garlic cloves, crushed
    2 tbsp olive oil
    juice of ½ lemon
    2 tsp tahini
    a pinch of cayenne pepper, plus extra to garnish
    sea salt

Put all the ingredients in a food processor or blender and blend
until smooth and creamy, adding a dash of water if necessary.
Check the flavour and adjust the seasoning according to
preference. Garnish with a little cayenne pepper and serve.

BABA GANOUSH

3GLs (140 calories per serving)
Serves 4

    1 tbsp olive oil
    2 garlic cloves, crushed
    ½ aubergine, cubed
    juice of ½ lemon
    25g sesame seeds
    25g fresh coriander
    115g live natural yogurt
    sea salt and ground black pepper

Heat the oil in a pan over medium heat and lightly fry the garlic for 2 minutes, then add the aubergine. Add 1 tbsp water to the pan, cover and steam-fry for 8 minutes or until soft.

Transfer to a food processor or blender and add the remaining ingredients, then blend until fairly smooth.

SMOKED SALMON PÂTÉ

5GLs (140 calories per serving)
Serves 4

   200g smoked salmon trimmings
   200g canned cannellini beans, drained and rinsed
   juice of 1 lemon
   a drizzle of olive oil, if needed
   1 tbsp chopped fresh dill
   sea salt and ground black pepper

Put all the ingredients in a food processor or blender and blend until the mixture is smooth, adding a little oil or water to loosen the mixture, if necessary. Chill before serving.

SPICED CHICKPEAS

5GLs (105 calories per serving)
Serves 3

   400g can chickpeas, drained and rinsed
   1 tsp olive oil

1 tbsp lemon juice
1 tsp paprika or cayenne pepper
sea salt and ground black pepper

Preheat the oven to 150°C/300°F/gas mark 2. Put the chickpeas in a bowl and add the oil. Toss well to coat, then tip into a baking tray and cook in the oven for 1 hour or until crisp, shaking the tray to move the chickpeas around from time to time.

Drizzle with lemon juice and sprinkle with paprika or cayenne pepper and seasoning.

Shake the chickpeas in the tray to coat thoroughly and then leave to cool.

GAZPACHO ANDALUZ

8GLs (100 calories per serving)
Serves 6

3 peppers (red, yellow and orange are the sweetest), chopped
1 cucumber, chopped
1 red onion, chopped
3 celery sticks, chopped
400g can chopped tomatoes
425ml tomato juice
2 garlic cloves, crushed
½ jar Peppadew sweet baby peppers, drained and chopped
sea salt and ground black pepper

Put half the fresh vegetables in a food processor or blender with the tomatoes, tomato juice and garlic, then blend until smooth.

Add the remaining vegetables and the Peppadew peppers, and season with black pepper. Serve.

CREAMY COLESLAW

3GLs (103 calories per serving)
Serves 6

    200g red or white cabbage, finely shredded
    90g carrots, grated
    ½ small onion, finely chopped
    1 tbsp low-fat mayonnaise
    1 tbsp low-fat live yoghurt or Greek yoghurt
    ground black pepper

Put all the ingredients into a bowl and mix thoroughly, then serve.

Recommended Reading

Patrick Holford, *The Low-GL Diet Bible*, Piatkus, 2009

Patrick Holford, *The Low-GL Diet Made Easy*, Piatkus, 2007

Patrick Holford and Fiona McDonald Joyce, *The Low-GL Diet Cookbook*, Piatkus, 2010

Patrick Holford and Fiona McDonald Joyce, *Food Glorious Food*, Piatkus, 2008

Patrick Holford & Jerome Burne, *Ten Secrets of Healthy Ageing*, Piatkus, 2012

Resources

Food

Chia seeds, the highest vegetarian source of omega-3, are available online and from www.totallynourish.com.

Lizi's Granola is available in most supermarkets and by mail order through www.totallynourish.com.

Patrick Holford's Get Up & Go low-GL, low-calorie shake provides all the nutrients needed for a nourishing low-GL meal, when blended with fruit and milk. Available from most good health food stores, Holland & Barrett and from online stores.

Sugar alternatives – xylitol Although it is best to avoid sugar and sugar alternatives as much as possible, there are two natural sugars that have the lowest GL score. These are blue agave syrup, which is used to sweeten healthier drinks, and xylitol. Xylitol has a GL score of one-seventh that of regular sugar and tastes the same. Therefore, if you need to sweeten a food or drink, use xylitol. It is available from some supermarkets and health food shops and also from www.totallynourish.com.

Exercise and weight loss

Resistance training equipment such as dumbbells are available at larger supermarkets.

Fitness Camp is an indoor/outdoor fitness camp set up by former Gladiator and athlete Kate Staples and decathlete Daley Thompson. For further information or to find a camp near you, see www.fitnesscamp.co.uk. Her trainers are also available through Zest4Life groups (see below). Kate also runs various retreats both in the UK and overseas.

Zest4Life is an exciting new and powerful health-improvement and weight-loss process designed to educate and motivate you to change and improve your body, your health and your well-being for good. The programmes are designed to create long-lasting change and are run by trained and qualified nutritional therapists, weight-loss coaches and fitness experts. Support can be provided in a variety of ways, depending on your time, budget and personal preferences. Choose from group weight loss, group health programmes, individual support, one-day transformation events, residential retreats, online coaching and well-being training courses.

The Zest4Life approach to nutrition is firmly grounded in learning how to eat healthily by balancing your blood sugar through following Patrick Holford's low-GL diet. Once you know the basics of good nutrition, you will be empowered to make the best choices for yourself and your family. You will feel better, have more energy and will maintain your success by continuing to eat this way as part of your everyday life.

The Zest4Life motivational coaching process for well-being and weight loss is one of the secrets to success: it helps you to overcome barriers and make changes so that it is easy and sustainable. The integration of metabolic boosting exercises, designed by leading fitness expert Kate Staples, completes the successful winning formula.

Contact Zest4Life via www.zest4life.com or call 0845 6039333.

Nutritional advice

Nutritional therapy To find a recommended nutritional therapist near you, visit the advice section on www.patrickholford.com. This service gives details on whom to see in the UK as well as internationally. If there is no one available nearby, you can always take an online assessment – see below.

Online 100% Health Programme Are you 100% healthy? Find out with our free health check and comprehensive personalised 100% Health Programme, giving you a personalised action plan, including diet and supplements.

Supplements

Finding your own perfect supplement programme can be confusing, but my website, www.patrickholford.com, offers useful guidance. The basic supplements – a high-strength multivitamin;

additional vitamin C; and an essential fat supplement containing omega-3 and omega-6 oils – can be bought as one supplement with GL Support – HCA (from tamarind), chromium and 5-HTP (tryptophan). This supplement combination for the low-GL diet is sold in daily strips in Patrick Holford's Optimum Nutrition Pack with GL Support. (Note: GL Support is sold as Appestop in South Africa.) Chromium, together with a high-potency cinnamon extract, is available as Cinnachrome.

CarboSlow, based on glucomannan fibre, is available in powder and capsule form. In the US, Canada and some other countries a fibre complex based on glucomannan is available as PGX.

Resveratrol Platinum, a high-potency resveratrol providing 125mg per capsule, is available from amazon.co.uk. Bioforte, providing 250mg of resveratrol, and Transmax, providing 500mg, are available from www.biotivia.co.uk.

Supplement suppliers

The following companies produce good-quality supplements that are widely available in the UK.

BioCare products are available at most health-food stores or visit www.biocare.com; tel.: 0121 433 3727.

Higher Nature Available at most independent health-food stores or visit www.highernature.co.uk; tel.: 0800 458 4747 (freephone within the UK)

Patrick Holford's range of daily supplement 'packs' are good for travelling or when you are away from home. Other supplements, including Get Up & Go and CarboSlow, are stocked by most good health-food stores, including Holland & Barrett – see www.hollandandbarrett.com. They are also available by mail order from www.totallynourish.com.

Solgar Available in most independent health-food stores, or visit www.solgar-vitamins.co.uk; tel.: +44 (0) 1442 890355.

Totally Nourish is an e-health shop that stocks many high-quality health products, including home test kits and supplements. Visit www.totallynourish.com; tel.: 0800 085 7749 (freephone within the UK).

Viridian For stockists, visit www.viridian-nutrition.com; tel.: +44 (0) 1327 878050.

And in other regions

Australia
Solgar supplements are available in Australia. Visit www.solgar.com.au; tel.: 1800 029 871 (free call) for your nearest supplier. Another good brand is Blackmores.

Kenya
Patrick Holford supplements are available in all Healthy U stores, www.healthy-U2000.com.

New Zealand

Patrick Holford products are available in New Zealand through Pacific Health, www.pachealth.co.nz; tel.: 0064 9815 0707.

Singapore

Patrick Holford and Solgar products are available in Singapore through Essential Living, www.essliv.com; tel.: 6276 1380.

South Africa

The original Patrick Holford vitamin and supplement brand from the UK is now available in South Africa through leading health-food stores, Dis-Chem and Clicks retail pharmacies. For more information on availability email info@holforddirect.co.za or contact 011 666 8994.

UAE

Patrick Holford supplements are available in Dubai and the UAE from Organic Foods & Café, www.organicfoodsandcafe.com; tel.: +971 44340577.

Notes

1 E. Lim, et al., 'Reversal of type 2 diabetes: Normalisation of beta cell function in association with decreased pancreas and liver triacyl-glycerol', *Diabetologia*, 2011 Oct;54(10):2506–14

2 J. Guevara-Aguirre, et al., 'Growth hormone receptor deficiency is associated with a major reduction in pro-aging signaling, cancer, and diabetes in humans', *Science Translational Medicine*, 2011;3(70):70ra13

3 H. Hirsch, et al., 'A transcriptional signature and common gene net-works link cancer with lipid metabolism and diverse human diseases', *Cancer Cell*, 2010;17(4):348–61

4 N. Cheng, et al., 'Follow-up survey of people in China with type 2 diabetes mellitus consuming supplemental chromium', *Journal of Trace Elements in Experimental Medicine*, 1999;12(2):55–60

5 E. Balk, et al., 'Effect of chromium supplementation on glucose metabolism and lipids: A systematic review of randomized controlled trials', *Diabetes Care*, 2007 Aug;30(8):2154–63

6 S. Anton et al., 'Effects of chromium picolinate on food intake and satiety', *Diabetes Technology and Therapeutics*, 2008 Oct;10(5):405–12

7 T. Ziegenfuss, et al., 'Effects of a Water-Soluble Cinnamon Extract on Body Composition and Features of the Metabolic Syndrome in Pre-Diabetic Men and Women', *Journal of the International Society of Sports Nutrition*, 2006; 3(2):45–53

8 R. Anson, et al., 'Intermittent fasting dissociates beneficial effects of dietary restriction on glucose metabolism and neuronal resistance to injury from calorie intake', *Proceedings of the National Academy of Sciences of the U.S.A.*, 2003;100(10):6216–20

9 J. Johnson, et al., 'Alternate day calorie restriction improves clinical findings and reduces markers of oxidative stress and inflammation in overweight adults with moderate asthma', *Free Radical Biology & Medicine*, 2007;42(5):665–74

10 K. Varady, et al., 'Improvements in body fat distribution and circulating adiponectin by alternate-day fasting versus calorie restriction', *Journal of Nutritional Biochemistry*, 2010;21(3):188–95

11 A. Hasegawa, et al., Department of Anesthesiology and Intensive Care Medicine, Oita University Faculty of Medicine, Yufu City, Oita, Japan, 'Alternate day calorie restriction improves systemic inflammation in a mouse model of sepsis induced by cecal ligation and puncture', *Journal of Surgical Research*, 2012 May 1;174(1):136–41

12 M. Klempel, et al., 'Alternate day fasting (ADF) with a high-fat diet produces similar weight loss and cardio-protection as ADF with a low-fat diet', *Metabolism*, 2012 Aug 10. [Epub ahead of print] PMID: 22889512

13 M. Klempel, et al., 'Intermittent fasting combined with calorie restriction is effective for weight loss and cardio-protection in obese women', *Nutrition Journal*, 2012 Nov 21;11(1):98

14 J. Lu, et al, 'Alternate day fasting impacts the brain insulin-signaling pathway of young adult male C57BL/6 mice', *Journal of Neurochemistry*, 2011 Apr;117(1):154–63

15 L. Castello, et al, 'Alternate-day fasting reverses the age-associated hypertrophy phenotype in rat heart by influencing the ERK and PI3K signaling pathways', *Mechanisms of Ageing Development*, 2011 Jun–Jul;132(6–7):305–14

16 I. Ahmet et al., 'Chronic alternate-day fasting results in reduced diastolic compliance and diminished systolic reserve in rats', *Journal of Cardiac Failure*, 2010 Oct;16(10):843–53.

17 M. Klempel, et al., 'Dietary and physical activity adaptations to alternate day modified fasting: Implications for optimal weight loss', *Nutrition Journal*, 2010 Sept 3;9:35

18 S. Bayod, et al., 'Long-term physical exercise induces changes in sirtuin 1 pathway and oxidative parameters in adult rat tissues', *Experimental Gerontology*, 2012 Dec;47(12):925–35

19 S. Bhutani, et al., 'Alternate-day fasting and endurance exercise combine to reduce body weight and favorably alter plasma lipids in obese humans', *Obesity* (Silver Spring), 2013 Feb 14, doi:10.1002/oby.20353. [Epub ahead of print]

20 R. Weiler, et al., 'Should health policy focus on physical activity rather than obesity? Yes', *British Medical Journal*, 2010;340:c2603

21 G. Reynolds, 'Phys Ed: How exercising keeps your cells young', *New York Times*, 2010 Jan. 27. Available at: http://well.blogs.nytimes.com/2010/01/27/phys-ed-how-exercising-keepsyour-cells-young/

22 J. Barger, et al., 'A low dose of dietary resveratrol partially mimics caloric restriction and retards aging parameters in mice', *Public Library of Sciences ONE* 2008;3(6): e2264.

Index

ageing hormone, *see* insulin
alternate-day fasting:
  downsides of 14–15
  easy to achieve 16
  explained 10–12
  and fast days, what to eat on
    46–54
  and fats 12–13
  and feast days, what to eat on
    54–5
  see also Alternate-Day Low-GL
    Diet; calorie restriction
Alternate-Day Low-GL Diet:
  days on and off 12
  eating less, living longer with 1–4
  with exercise 17
  frequently asked questions about
    17–20
  history behind 1–21
  recipes, *see* recipes and dishes
  see also alternate-day fasting
Atkins diet 7, 25
Atkins, Dr Robert 25

breakfast:
  on fast days 47–8
  low-GL 33
  recipes for 47–8

Caenorhabditis elegans 4
calorie restriction (CR) 2–4

  see also alternate-day fasting
carbohydrate:
  balancing 31–2
  eating fat and protein with 25–6
  foods containing, listed 32
  see also glycemic load
cardio training 40–1
  see also exercise
case studies:
  Ellie xv
  Wendy 16
chromium 8–9
cinnamon 9–10
'CRonies' 2

Diabetes Care 9
diet-and-exercise workout in
    practice 44–58
  and fast days, what to eat on
    46–54
  and feast days, what to eat on
    54–5
  typical weekly routine 45
dishes, *see* recipes and dishes
drinks, best 56

Ecuador dwarves 7
exercise:
  Alternate Reverse Lunge 66
  best time for, and eating 56
  boosting diet with 35–43

Box Press with Alternate Leg Lift 68
calf stretches 75
cardio training 40–1, 59–60; *see also* exercise: routines, explained and discussed
cool-down 75
with diet, in practice, *see* diet-and-exercise workout in practice
enjoying 41
Full Push-up 72
and gene switching 17
good for body 37
hamstring stretches 75
interval training 41–2
Jumping Squats 71
Modified Box Press 64
Mountain Climbers 73
Pendulum Lunge 74
Plank Jacks 69
Plank Step-outs 65
quad stretch 76
resistance/strength training 38–9, 60; *see also* exercise: routines, explained and discussed
Reverse Lunge with Triceps Kick-back 70
routines, explained and discussed 59–76
Squat Shoulder Press 67
time and equipment for 61
Wall Sit 63
warm-up 62

fats, and alternate-day fasting 12–13

genes:
Foxo 6
Grim Reaper 5, 6, 7, 24
'skinny' 4–5, 11–12, 13, 18, 47, 57

Sweet Sixteen 5
glycemic load:
breakfasts low in 33
explained 22, 26–8
and foods, listed 27–8
golden rules concerning 25–6
model meal 29–30
snacks low in 34
see also carbohydrate
goal, reaching, what to do then 58

Holly, Prof. Jeff 5

IGF-1 7
insulin:
as ageing hormone 5–6
chromium and cinnamon to lower 8–10
ill health's connection with 7–8
sensitivity to, importance of 23–4
sensitivity to, improving 8
interval training 41–2
see also exercise

Kenyon, Prof. Cynthia 4, 5
Klempel, Monica 12

Mattson, Dr Mark 11

protein, options 31

recipes and dishes:
apple, spiced 48
Apple and Tuna Salad 49, 78
Baba Ganoush 91–2
Beany Vegetable Soup 50, 80–1
Butternut Squash Salad 49
Chestnut and Butterbean Soup 50, 81
Chickpea and Spinach Curry 52, 86–7
cod, roasted 52

recipes and dishes – *continued*
  Creamy Coleslaw 94
  eggs 48
  Feta Salad 50
  Garlic Chilli Prawns with Pak
    Choi 52, 87–8
  Gazpacho Anadaluz 93–4
  Get Up & Go 47–8
  granola 48
  High-energy Lentil Soup 51,
    83–4
  Homemade Hummus 91
  Indian Spiced Chicken 51
  kipper 48
  Lentil and Lemon Soup 50,
    81–2
  Mexican Bean Dip 90
  omelette 52
  Pasta with Borlotti Bolognese 51,
    85–6
  Peruvian Quinoa Salad 49
  porridge 48
  Quick Pea and Mint Soup 51,
    84–5
  Quinoa Tabbouleh 50, 79–80
  salads 49–50, 78–80
  Salmon Fillets with New Potatoes
    52–3, 88–9
  salmon, steamed 52
  Salmon-Stuffed Avocado 49
  Smoked Salmon Pâté 92
  soups 50–1, 80–5
  Spiced Chickpeas 92–3
  Spicy Pumpkin and Tofu Soup
    51, 82–3
  Trout with Puy Lentils and
    Roasted Tomatoes on the
    Vine 53, 89–90
  Walnut and Three-bean Salad 49,
    78–9
  yoghurt with berries 48
resistance/strength training 38–9
  see also exercise
resources:
  exercise and weight loss 98–9
  food 97
  nutrition 99
  other regions 101–2
  supplements 99–101

salads:
  on fast days 49–50
  recipes for 49–50, 78–80
'skinny genes' 4–5, 13, 18, 47, 57
snacks:
  on fast days 53–4
  low-GL 34
soups:
  on fast days 50–1
  recipes for 50–1, 80–5
strength training, *see*
    resistance/strength training
sugar:
  alternatives to 29
  breaking habit of 28–9
supplements:
  recommended 57, 99–100
  suppliers of 100–1

vegetables:
  non-starchy 32–3
  starchy 27

Walford, Roy 2–4

Zest4Life v, xiii, 77, 98–9

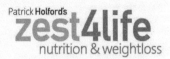
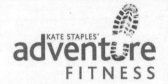
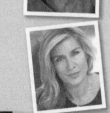
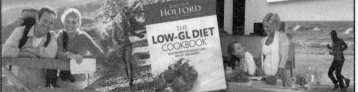

Six weeks to a slimmer you!

You don't have to be a saint every day!

A slimmer, healthier, happier you with our Six Weeks to Success programme

Top nutrition expert, Patrick Holford, guides you through the most effective way to control your weight, burn fat and regain your health and energy. **Top exercise expert, Kate Staples**, shows you how to do the least exercise for the most fat-burning effect, and one of Patrick's **top nutrition coaches** guides you week-by-week on the most effective and easy to follow diet, helping you avoid the usual pitfalls and also to keep you motivated.

Here's what you get, and why:

How to Lose Weight the GL Way - watch this 45 minute film of Patrick explaining exactly why his low GL diet is the best way to both control your weight, burn fat and regain your health and energy.

The Best Exercises to Burn Fat - watch and participate in this fat burning session with leading exercise guru, Kate Staples, as she shows you how to burn fat, lose inches and gain fatburning muscle.

Six Weeks to Success Workbook - this will become your bible, giving clear instructions on what to do, week by week, including how to implement Patrick's new Alternate Day Low GL approach. You will also monitor your progress using a range of tools included in the workbook.

My 50 favourite low GL recipes - these downloadable recipes are the easiest to make and most delicious, as chosen by hundreds of successful low GL dieters.

Six Online Coaching sessions - these can be accessed at any time, from anywhere in the World, all you need is an internet connection. They will provide practical support to help you to meet your goals.

You can have all this and more in our Six Weeks to Success programme, giving you all the resources in your living room for six weeks.

Join today at www.patrickholford.com/six_weeks

Also you will receive a **free six month membership** to Patrick Holford's 100% Health Club, giving you instant access to his bi-monthly newsletters, hundreds of Special Reports on key health issues and blog discussions.